Curing Food Allergies and Common Illnesses

Curing Food Allergies and Common Illnesses

Parasitic Micro—Organisms and Your Health

Alan Hunter D.Dt.

Ashgrove Publishing
London and Bath

CONTENTS

Acknowledgements

I wish to thank the following, either for their direct or indirect contributions to this book, or for the influence their work has had on my views on the cause of illness.

Willowdeen Shelton, of San Antonio, Texas, for allowing me access to her father, Dr. Herbert Shelton's work. Dr. Shelton's wonderful writings on natural health and fasting have played a major part in my research for this book.

Charlotte Gerson, of the Gerson Institute in California, for contributing case histories from the Gerson therapy. Her father, Dr. Max Gerson, devised the Gerson dietary therapy, which has saved the lives of thousands. His work has also been extremely important in my reaching the conclusions contained in this book.

Dr. Hulda Clark, of California, whose works on parasitic micro-organisms inspired me to return to a subject I had pushed aside.

Dr. Virginia Vetrano, of Barksdale, Texas, a colleague of Dr. Shelton, who kindly gave me permission to use her delightful story 'Tosca's fever'.

Keki Sidhwa N.D., D.O., of England, and Dr. William Esser, of Florida, under both of whom I have fasted and whose libraries of rare books on natural healing ensured my stays were not only a delight, but highly educational. I also thank Keki for his contribution to this book.

I also wish to thank the following for their permissions to quote: Professor Anthony Milton of the Department of Pharmacology, University of Cambridge; Magdalena Hanich of Springer-Verlag, Heidelberg, West Germany, for permission to quote from *Pyretics and Antipyretics*; Arlene Phalon of W.W. Norton & Co., New York, for excerpts from *Biological Science*; Carole Goodall of Arnold Publishers, London, for information from *Microbial and Parasitic Infection*; Prof. A.D. Charters of Kalamunda, Western Australia, for excerpts from *Human Parasitology*; Sarah McCrae of Blackwell Science, Oxford, for permission to quote from *Modern Parasitology*; and Prof. Robert Forman of New York for the list of food allergy symptoms taken from *How to Control Your Allergies*.

1.

The Search for a Cure

To recover from a chronic illness is rare. Most sufferers, once they contract the disease, will live their entire lives under the limitations imposed by their complaint. They may see the symptoms fluctuate, have good and bad days, but their illness will always return to haunt them.

The family doctor will do his best, but his treatment will almost invariably consist of drugs to alleviate the symptoms. Welcome though such relief may be, once the drugs wear off the condition will be as bad as ever, if not worse.

The information in this book will give *real* hope to sufferers of chronic disease. The book contains a new discovery about illness and presents information which can lead to an actual cure for a host of common illnesses for which medical science presently has no answer.

What you will read is in advance of conventional medical wisdom, insofar as it describes an original and unique method of health recovery, one which doesn't simply target the symptoms, but shows the *cause* of many common health disorders and, moreover, supplies an actual *solution*.

If you are one of the millions of silent sufferers, taking daily medication but in truth getting no better, then please read this book.

There may also appear to be a strong 'food allergy' angle to this book. Do not let that put you off, as it is almost certainly entirely relevant to your recovery from illness.

I will be able to show that, no matter what your complaint, there is almost certainly a dietary connection of which you are probably unaware. If you have any of the symptoms listed in Chapter 15, this book will almost certainly give you a new insight into your illness, as well as providing you with a totally original solution!

For the past fifteen years I have seen clients with all manner of health problems who never even considered that there might be a food link to their illness. I have been able to show nearly all of them that there most certainly was a connection. Making the tie-in can be enormously difficult unless you know how.

I, too, was a patient. My own illness spurred me on to a 30 year search for the answer. My experience followed the sequence of events with which many sufferers are now familiar: the initial appearance of illness; no help from the family doctor other than the offer of drugs; continuation of the illness despite years of such drug-taking; and the wonderful, unexpected discovery that all the time there was a diet link to my illness that no one had even considered!

It really doesn't matter what your illness is, there is a strong chance that there will be a dietary link. If so, you will then find yourself joining the growing world-wide band of 'food allergics'. These are simply people with ordinary illnesses who have managed, by their own endeavours, to find the diet connection.

It is estimated that over 80% of people sitting in doctors' surgeries have what are referred to as 'masked food allergies', which can be responsible for their ill health. Yet these people almost always come out of the surgery with a prescription for drugs which can actually worsen their long-term outlook. They will most likely have been given no hint at all by the doctor that what they are eating can be responsible for their symptoms. For, unbelievably, doctors get no training in the subject. And because some doctors feel embarrassed at having missed a powerful tool for influencing their patients' health, many are hostile to the very suggestion that diet can play a part.

Most doctors are reluctant to accept that the answer to so many common health problems can lie on the dinner plate. They recognise that ill health, even death, can result from putting other substances into that hole in your head: for example alcohol (liver disease), tobacco (heart disease, circulatory disease, and cancers). Yet they appear to have overlooked the possibility that the largest load of material you will ever push into your body might just play a part in your health.

But whilst doctors grind through their daily practices blissfully unaware of the food link to illness, it hasn't escaped vets. Take an ill snake, for example, to a vet, and one of the first things he will ask is 'And what are you feeding it?'.

But the quality of your diet and your overall health is only one part of the equation. The specific linking of foods to your actual symptoms is the other. When that occurs, we can make that patient aware of the diet link and he will then recognise for the first time that he is a food allergic.

Regardless of a doctor's training, the association between diet and symptoms has been so soundly recorded over the last 30 or so years, in thousands of books and articles on food allergies, that it would take a brave – or truly ignorant – doctor to refute that there can be a connection.

Even those practitioners who do know how to diagnose the food allergy condition have only been able so far to assist patients in identifying their troublesome foods and then advising them to avoid these dietary substances.

It has always been my personal goal to uncover not only the *reason* people become ill in such a fashion, but also to find the cure for the condition. Whilst the vast majority of patients and, indeed, practitioners, aspire to identify the culprit foods and other substances in order to avoid them, in my view that simply does not go far enough. To find the actual cause of 'food allergies' has always been my objective.

Although patients will admit to immense satisfaction when they identify specific foods or drinks that can bring on an attack of their symptoms, that is only going half way. The reason they are like that in the first place has been given little attention. And certainly the cure has never been found. Until now.

It has taken me *thirty years*, but I have now done just that. I have found the answer to the food allergy condition. As the syndrome has been linked to so many other health disorders this solution serves also to explain the cause of many other medical conditions. I contend that these include arthritis, depression, fatigue and a veritable catalogue of 'everyday' disorders, as exhibited in Chapter 15.

Furthermore, the answer I give is so packed with common sense that even sceptical doctors, untrained in the subject of food allergies, would be hard pressed to find fault with it - although I am sure many will try!

I will also show you that the food/chemical allergy condition is linked to parasites within your body, most specifically at the site of your symptom. And that these parasites exist within you as a result of long term poor diet, in either yourself, your parents, or both. Furthermore I have come up with a surprising reason why these micro-organisms will want to settle inside *you* and not someone else!

2.

My Illness Appears

As a young man I was a superbly fit judo player, being selected to represent Great Britain in international matches and ranked No.3 in Europe at Under-21 level. I never became ill and couldn't for a moment understand why anyone else did. Whilst friends of the same age hurtled headlong into the usual merry-go-round of late nights, drinking, clubs, and girlfriends, I wasn't that 'weak.' I had better things to do.

But it wasn't to last. At the relatively elderly age of 20 I succumbed to the attractions that I had so stoically avoided. It wasn't long before I, too, was burning the candle at both ends. But instead of lighting the wick with the relative calmness of a match, I was using a blow-torch. If I had foregone the pleasures of teenage years before, I sure was about to make up for it.

Before long, the addictive personality that I had undoubtedly inherited from my alcoholic father was to surface. From being a committed and dedicated sportsman, it wasn't long before I was indulging in drinking, night-life, and that phenomenon of the 60's youth scene, street drugs galore.

From the introductory weekends of casual drinking and dancing, the progression into advanced hedonistic pleasures was pursued at almost breakneck speed. Before long, drugs such as 'purple hearts', 'black bombers' and 'dex', were becoming part of my daily diet. The yo-yoing of emotion, from the heights of supreme confidence to the depths of despair, was becoming a familiar theme in my search for perpetual pleasure.

After a mere couple of years on this self-destructive course, I became ill for the first time in my life. Fatigue, a condition totally alien to me, now became a familiar companion. I had periods of unclear thinking, my short term memory was affected and my attention span poor. I had a mild sort of depression: not true depression I considered, but more than the average experience of 'feeling blue'. I retained an excellent sense of humour, but whilst I knew I still had this side to my personality, the despair of the illness masked it. It was also highly unpredictable. I would never know when the feeling would come over me. I could be chirpy one minute and then feel awful the next.

However, like everyone else, I had absolute faith in my doctor. At the start of my illness I had not the slightest clue that my lifestyle could be contributing to my new found state of ill health. And neither did he.

All he could do was treat my symptoms with drugs. He would give me medication for my fatigue and something for the 'depression'. And, though they gave short-term relief, they did nothing to remove the cause. As soon as the drugs wore off, the symptoms returned. Because the cause was not being addressed, my slide into even poorer health was inexorable.

When my doctor eventually told me that there was nothing else he could do, I was devastated. I certainly considered suicide. If my doctor could not help then, surely, I reasoned, I was destined for a life of misery.

But the single-mindedness that had served me well in sport was thankfully not to desert me. I was determined to beat the condition. My fight back started with a visit to the library…

A fascinating book

It took several weeks, flitting from one health topic to another, before I hit on the particular book that was to be the turning point in my life. That book, although I didn't know it at the time, was to keep me alive. It was to show me that there was something that the doctor had missed, but that I could now do for myself.

The book was called *Nutrition and Your Mind,* by a Californian, Dr. George Watson. In it he showed that many patients with illnesses, both physical and mental, for which their doctor could find no explanation, could have a food link. Their symptoms could be turned on and off by items in their diet! This was absolutely astonishing. Certainly, if what I was reading was true, it simply begged the question as to why it wasn't being applied world wide, so saving millions from misery.

Then I began to realise how embarrassed doctors and psychiatrists would be that they had overlooked such a 'simple' explanation. Self-interest and self-protection would play no small part in their resistance.

After all, if you had been studying for years at medical school, not knowing the cause of most illnesses, trained to dish out drugs to temporarily alleviate symptoms, would you want to be told you were barking up the wrong tree? Would you want to learn that something you had no training in, something as simple as food, could be responsible for most of the common disorders you were treating on a daily basis and for which you had no answer? Somehow I don't think you would.

I could hardly be prised away from Dr. Watson's book. It all began to fall into place. Here was something new (it was in the 1960s), something revolutionary, and something which made eminent sense. Not only that, but something tangible, something that one could quickly eliminate or confirm as being relevant. Dr. Watson told of one patient with depression who had spent thousands of dollars on psychoanalysis, years on the couch being quizzed about her childhood, only to have her depression lift dramatically after allergenic foods were removed from her diet.

Many things in the book suggested to me that I was on the right track. And if my doctor was ensconced in old teachings, then so be it; it certainly wasn't going to stop me investigating this new food allergy phenomenon.

I travel to Rome

Before long I was writing to Dr. Watson, asking to come over and be tested. The food allergy condition was unknown in the U.K. at that time and certainly there was no one in Britain able to test. He wrote back saying that there was someone nearer than California and I could go to them. I had hoped that would mean the U.K., but it turned out to be Italy, in that most beautiful of cities, Rome. Soon I was on my way to the Eternal City to be tested.

It was pointed out to me that it was almost certainly the substances most regularly 'consumed', that is, the foods, drinks, alcohol, even cigarettes, that would prove to be the factors responsible for my ill health, if indeed any link were to be found. My favourite drink was tea, of which I would have at least 20 cups a day.

The Italian doctor asked his nurse to take my blood pressure before and after each test substance, in order to compare readings. A major change, up or down, signified 'allergy' to the substance tested.

The actual food or drink being tested was not divulged to the patient, lest it provoked a psychological response. However, if I had been told I was being tested for tea, I would comfortably and confidently have predicted that it wouldn't have had the slightest adverse affect on me. After all, I loved tea. If it had been causing me harm, believe me, I would have known! But I did not know that the foods you love very often prove to be the problem ones. The connection is never as easy to make as you would expect.

On the day of the tea test, the nurse took my blood pressure. Then I was told to sample the test substance. The method used was the old-fashioned 'sniff testing'. I felt no change whatsoever in my condition, and a few minutes later, she took my blood pressure again.

I watched her puzzled expression as she took it. She appeared to consider that the equipment, the sphygmomanometer, was faulty, so she tried again. She then called a male nurse over. He too took my blood pressure. Now they both looked baffled. It turned out that my blood pressure post-test had dropped to a dangerously low level, yet I had felt nothing. So my beloved tea became one of the first substances to which I was shown to be 'allergic'.

A later test was memorable. After sniffing the substance, I slumped over the table, disorientated. I was not unconscious, but I was certainly out of it, unaware of the blood pressure readings. This highly allergic reaction was to another substance that I took on a regular basis. A food? No. It was tobacco!

I had fallen into the common trap of becoming a relatively heavy cigarette smoker by that time, never considering for a moment that the 4,000 (yes, four thousand) chemicals in each cigarette might be playing a part in my condition. First tea, now cigarettes: it seemed as if life's pleasures were being denied me, one by one. With enormous difficulty I managed to stop smoking for a few days, but then succumbed again. During these few days my symptoms lifted considerably; I felt much better. However, within thirty seconds of inhaling, my familiar symptoms returned with a vengeance!

For the first time, I had made a connection between the puzzling symptoms of my illness (that had completely baffled my doctors), and something I was putting into my mouth. It was truly enlightening. I was thrilled with the discovery. I now had a degree of control over my illness that had thus far eluded me. I was exhilarated!

After spending a month in Rome as a house guest of the doctor, I returned to Britain with a decidedly different slant on my health problem. Although I arrived back in Britain with more knowledge than when I left, the information I had collected was, I later realised, extremely primitive. But I had enough to be getting on with. I had made the connection.

At first, this connection between my symptoms and foods or drinks was relatively easy to make. But, frustratingly, it appeared that more and more substances in my diet were affecting me. I would avoid one substance that provoked my symptoms, only to find other foods taking its place. This happens with some food allergics. Whilst many prove allergic to only a few substances, others can become ill from virtually everything they eat, drink or even inhale.

As cigarette smoke was my main allergen (the substance to which I was allergic), and because tobacco is powerfully addictive, this proved to be the most difficult substance of all to give up. It took me years finally to wrench myself free.

As I eliminated problem foods from my diet, previously innocent foods would begin to produce reactions. I was 'reacting' to almost everything. It appeared that no matter what I put in my mouth, it would bring on my symptoms. Frustrating is the only word which comes near to how I felt, but it doesn't truly describe the despair I faced on a daily basis in my battle to recover.

I read every book I could get hold off on the subject, most of which were American. It was clear that if doctors could miss something so obvious and omnipresent as food, then they might have missed a whole lot more. I read as much as I could on every related discipline, from 'classical' dietetics to 'classical' allergy, from single nutrient deficiencies to complex deficiency syndromes, from Enzyme Therapy to Amino Acids, Naturopathy to Kinesiology, Natural Therapeutics to Megavitamin Therapy, Fasting to Nature Cure, Natural Hygiene to Orthopathy, Kirlian Photography to Pyrexia, Electro-physiology to the Gerson Therapy, and too many more even to mention. I was seeking and obtaining books and information from the 1700s to the present day on every subject relating to diet and illness. I was contacting out-of-print booksellers for reprints of old books on all and any allied subjects. My appetite, if you like, for the subject, was insatiable.

I stop eating altogether

After struggling with my diet for many years, I had to acknowledge that I was now at the stage where virtually everything I was putting into my body was bringing about a reaction, so I turned to fasting as a possible solution to my problem.

The books I had on Therapeutic Fasting were littered with case histories of people achieving recovery from a variety of health problems. It seemed a reasonably logical progression for someone who became ill upon eating everything, to begin to eat nothing. The recoveries quoted in these books inevitably occurred after long fasts. And by that I mean upwards of 30 days, with one as long as 103 days.

Therapeutic fasting means eating nothing at all and drinking only pure water – as much as thirst demands. If you hear of someone being put on a juice fast, they should more properly be described as being on a juice *diet*.

I experimented much with fasting. I would fast in my house for four days before succumbing to what were probably imaginary, but certainly powerful, cravings. I would fast at another time for six days, then again for seven, and so on. The length of each fast depended on my ability to ride out the inevitable cravings that existed at the beginning.

Whilst it is commonly observed that all hunger disappears after 48 hours, I would regularly find myself having brief but horrendous cravings many days into the fast. And it took some considerable skill to recognise that, if I didn't give in to these seemingly immovable longings, they would ultimately pass.

My seven day fasts were later followed by others of 10 days, then 11, 12,14, and the occasional 16 day fast. But whilst I was most definitely experiencing improvement in symptoms some of the time, it was never lasting.

The cravings that would come over me were horrendous and I consider them being not unlike those encountered by someone on heroin undergoing 'cold turkey'. Certainly they could be likened to the powerful urges to smoke which a smoker experiences when he attempts to give up.

The logic behind therapeutic fasting is that all animals in nature automatically stop eating when they become ill. Injured animals will seek isolation and shelter and cease eating whilst awaiting recovery. They will drink water but will not resume eating until they are well – and that includes waiting for a broken limb to heal!

I wanted to do a long fast, that is upwards of 40 days. I knew the only way to do so would be to go to a clinic. But fasting clinics, where they carry out true fasts, were few and far between. I found the only experienced fasting practitioner in Britain, Keki Sidhwa, a naturopath who had visited and learned from the world's most knowledgeable fasting expert, Dr. Herbert Shelton. Dr. Shelton had a doctorate in physiology and the experience he had gained over many years in fasting thousands of patients with all kinds of disorders, was unique. His knowledge of what happens in the human body, when eating ceases completely, was unsurpassed.

I went to Keki's home in the south of England to begin my fast. I was fasted for 30 days. This was a longer fast than he commonly supervised at his home and as his family were coming from India to visit, I had little choice but to curtail the experiment prematurely. I know that I was in the frame of mind on that thirtieth day to carry the fast to forty days or much longer, but I had to end it when requested by Keki, as it could be dangerous to carry it beyond that time without proper supervision.

My symptoms on day 30 were not vastly improved. But oddly enough, when I started eating, my symptoms did improve – remarkably. And that improvement lasted for several days. But within a few days more, I was back to the familiar symptoms of illness.

After many more shorter fasts, I eventually tried a long fast at home. To ensure success I locked myself in my house and threw the key out of the window to my daughter. At the time I was divorced, otherwise I am sure my wife would have had something to say about being unable to get out of the house!

I lasted 28 days before caving in to a fleeting but overwhelming craving for, of all things, tomatoes. Experience now tells me that this craving was almost certainly a false one. It was, I'm sure, a clever self-delusory ruse to return me to my old addictive eating habits. By expressing a desire to eat a 'healthy' food such as tomatoes, I was giving myself permission to return to eating *per se*, indirectly giving me access to the foods I really wanted – the processed foods that virtually all of us in modern society crave. And as I knew I would react to virtually everything, even healthy foods, I often thought 'what the heck', and would indulge in less nutritious, but certainly tasty, food.

A further 21 day fast in America was later to follow, but my return to the addictive eating of wrong foods was a common consequence of such self-imposed discipline. I would 'reward' myself after going without any food for such a long time, with a return to compulsive eating. It appeared that I was truly a person of extremes; in virtually every facet of my life I would oscillate from one extreme to the other. If I wasn't indulging in alcohol to excess, I moved on to foods and excelled in that area too. Then I would go to the very opposite end of the scale and eat absolutely nothing. This pattern of extreme eating stayed with me for a long time, as my experimentation in diet continued.

Although I tried many fasts, none of them fully brought me to recovery. However, I sincerely feel that because of the length of my illness (30 years) a truly long fast would have been required to achieve lasting success. Whilst many people make astonishing recoveries from illness after fasting for only a few weeks, the more chronic amongst us often require longer. However fasting is something that should *never* be undertaken without proper supervision.

3.

An Early and Fascinating Observation

It was not long into my illness before I realised my symptoms were permanent. I was reacting to all foods and was virtually never free from the symptoms that I had come to detest. I would go to sleep with them and wake up with them. They were with me effectively 24 hours a day.

A few years after first developing this condition, by now identified as 'food allergic', I developed a fever. I had never been prone to getting high temperatures, and, in fact, over the past thirty years, I have only ever had four. During the fever, I made an odd, but decidedly welcome observation. Whilst I had the high temperature, my familiar hated symptoms of food allergy deserted me. My food allergy symptoms had entirely disappeared!

Although I was feeling grim, with the general malaise that accompanies fever, the 'food allergy' symptoms that I knew so very well had completely cleared. I was totally free from my illness. It was a wonder to behold and there was no explanation for it. I remember remarking to my wife that my symptoms had left. But this happy occasion was not to last. As soon as my fever left, my symptoms returned.

I knew there had to be a clue to the origins of my illness in that fever. High temperature, fever, and the absence of symptoms just had to be linked; but try as I might, I could not fathom how. I went back to the medical library to read up on fever - pyrexia - but the information was so vast, and yet by the admission of the highly-qualified medical authors so incomplete, that I couldn't put my recovery down to any one specific mechanism.

A further three periods of fever, each separated by several years, were to follow. And without exception, when the fever was present, my symptoms entirely disappeared! It was certainly no exaggeration to say that I positively welcomed a fever after the first experience. Since that time I have spoken with many food allergy sufferers, with a wide variety of symptoms. They confirmed that they too experienced a welcome release from their condition during fever.

I had no doubt that whatever mechanism was occurring in me during these times of fever would hold the key to the food allergy condition.

4.

Analysing the 'Allergic' Condition

(*Including Temperature Charts*)

I would often sit down and think about my illness. I tried to do the seemingly impossible: to work out through logic just what was going on in my body. What brought about these symptoms and how could they then be influenced by incoming foods or chemical factors? I would invariably end up going round in circles and so would give up analysing and return to 'normal' living.

I then began to study dietetics, and to see people with health problems that might be linked to the food allergy condition. I was helping these people achieve the recognition that what they were consuming was contributing to their symptoms. Patients were extremely grateful for this insight into their illness, as it was an awareness that had been denied them by their doctors, who had not been trained in the subject.

However, I was unhappy that in merely assisting people to find the food link to their disorders I was not doing enough. I desperately wanted to discover just why people, including myself, were 'allergic' and suffering in the first place. Why were some allergic and others not? I made it my goal to find out.

On one occasion when I was again analysing my condition, I seemed to move a step further than I had previously. I found myself examining aspects of the phenomenon I had never previously considered . . .

It was standard practice, in all the books on food and chemical allergies, effectively to warn people off processed foods. Most authorities on the subject were of the opinion it was the additives in tinned foods that were responsible for triggering the food allergic's symptoms. Most of the tinned, packaged, bottled and other processed foods on supermarket shelves have some sort of adulterants in them. Clinical ecologists - those doctors and therapists who recognise and treat the food allergy condition - point to the vast number of chemical constituents as being responsible for any accentuation in the patients' symptoms.

But my own experience suggested there was more to that than was first supposed. I, for one, reacted to foods that were totally organic and uncontaminated.

The Gerson Therapy belies the 'additives' theory

The Gerson Therapy is a dietary approach to illness, most notably cancer; but it has also had tremendous success in treating a large number of other disorders. In effect it simply consists of eating foods that are natural and uncontaminated by modern food processing methods. Considerable evidence has been gathered to show that by following such a strict but natural eating regimen, all manner of health problems can be overcome. A German doctor, Max Gerson, had adapted an old Italian dietary approach to migraine for his own patients with the condition. Not only did many of his patients recover from their migraines, they also noticed the disappearance of other symptoms.

The diet was simple and natural: no tinned foods, no packaged foods, no alcohol, no tobacco, and so on. Boring though that might sound, it was eagerly embraced by those patients who were utterly desperate for help and would do anything in the hope of recovering.

As the Gerson Therapy, as it was later to be called, became better and better known, so the number of documented recoveries from all manner of illnesses increased. However, Gerson's ability to succeed where orthodox medicine had failed didn't go down well with the medical establishment.

Aware that the embarrassed medical profession would grasp at any reason to denounce these safest-of-all approaches to health recovery, Dr. Gerson insisted that those patients who were diagnosed with cancer have this diagnosis confirmed by outside hospitals. There could then be no later accusation of results being 'doctored' when patients were restored to health. Many of these patients had been sent home to die with supposedly 'incurable' cancers but recovered and lived for 20, 30 or even 40 years after experiencing the Gerson Therapy.

Having read all about the Gerson Therapy, I recognised a curious fact: as well as cancers, many of these patients had secondary conditions such as depression, arthritis, insomnia, and a host of common symptoms normally recognised to be of 'food allergy' origin. Not only did the cancer clear up, so did their other symptoms.

No consideration of food allergy was taken into account by any of the Gerson doctors in applying their dietary approach. They barged ahead with their wide and varied fruit and vegetable diet, yet the patients would still recover from their ills. Many of these patients would doubtless have been diagnosed as 'allergic' if proper investigation had been carried out.

Notwithstanding, I considered that applying a natural-diet approach such as the Gerson therapy to a food allergic individual should make considerable sense. After all, if all these patients, who had symptoms identical to the food allergic, could recover, it seemed highly probable that the only reason they were not labelled 'food allergics' in the first place was simply because they hadn't been tested; that the allergy condition had never been considered.

The Gerson Therapy is quite a difficult regimen to follow, consisting almost totally of fruits and vegetables. As any 'civilised' person would acknowledge, a dramatic shift from the usual addictive, processed diet to such a relatively spartan one would require considerable stoicism and the ability to 'ride out' overwhelming cravings. The diet does however have one redeeming factor - homemade vegetable soup is most positively permitted. Made from organically grown vegetables, such a welcome hot meal compensates wonderfully for an otherwise mostly raw diet.

Allergic to everything!

In an attempt to recover from my own long-standing food allergy condition, I would often commence the Gerson therapy, only to abandon it several months later - far short of the normal period recommended for recovery of 18 months to 3 years – because every food item on the diet was making me ill. After these failed attempts, I would often resort to not eating at all – fasting.

I recorded in my diary, however, that despite the seeming setbacks the Gerson therapy produced, I had quite a number of extremely well days, which I had never before experienced (except when I had a fever). I also had experiences, when on the therapy, of reduced reactions. In other words, the reaction I was having today was considerably reduced from the reaction I had yesterday. Such insights into the likely pattern of recovery were encouraging. But as these good periods were inevitably followed by long days of despair, the inspiration was knocked out of me and I would abandon the diet sooner or later.

I recognised that it wasn't just processed foods, with all the chemical adulterants they contain, that could bring about my food allergy symptoms. Those Clinical Ecologists who were suggesting that it was the sprays on the vegetables that might be causing the return of symptoms, or the chemical constituents in packaged foods, were getting it only half right. What about people like me, who would experience full-blown symptoms eating organically grown fruits? That appeared to blow the entire additives-causing food-allergic symptoms to smithereens.

Subnormal body temperature

I was aware that I did have a lower than normal body temperature. Whilst the normal is 98.6 degrees. F., I would regularly read my morning temperature as in the high 96s and low to mid 97s.

It is also well known that a body temperature reduced even by a single degree can cause a host of symptoms, mental as well as physical. It is estimated that upwards of 40% of the population of the entire United States has a subnormal core body temperature.[1] Such a large percentage of people with compromised body temperatures will almost certainly be mirrored in other industrialised countries around the world.

It was very interesting however to note that on one seven-month attempt at the Gerson Therapy, there was an erratic but definite improvement in my morning temperature readings. I would note more and more days of higher temperature readings as well as more and more episodes of several days of higher readings strung together.

I recorded my morning temperatures throughout that seven-month period, and the gradual but unyielding climb in my body temperature was to play a critical part several years later when I was to discover the actual cause of food allergies. Here is that chart:

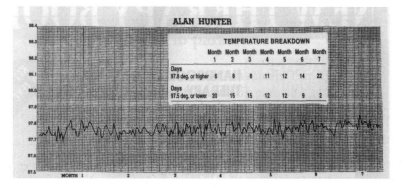

Dwelling once more on the fact that I could react to such natural foods as organic fruits and vegetables, something which I had always known reared its head again, but this time with a new pair of specs... It was the familiar realisation that the fault was not with the fruits or vegetables, it was with me.

Whilst I had known this for many years, it was something one tended not to dwell on. This time however, it demanded to be addressed. It wasn't enough merely advising patients to avoid processed foods because these foods contained contaminants. What was it in people like me who react to foods that are uncontaminated?

If I were to avoid all the dietary substances that brought on my symptoms, I would undoubtedly die from starvation. What fault within me made me react to the foods Nature apparently intended me to eat?

Nature intended man to eat natural foods such as fruits. If I was 'reacting' to them, then the fault surely lay not with the fruits but within me. Advancing that thought, the fault not only had to be within me, but within me surely, at the site of the symptom.

I considered that as every food allergic's symptoms are unique to them, then each patient would have his own particular spot in the body where the problem occurred. If it were depression or irritability for example, the head area would be the one with the problem; and if it was arthritis in the knee, then the knee was the problem site. Whatever the symptom, the same area in that patient's body would react over and over again.

I consider the options

Taking the logic one step further, if the fault within the patient is at the site of the symptom, then there has to be an unnatural process at work at that site.

There could only be, I reasoned, three options. There was:

1. Something damaged at the site of the symptom
   or
2. Something missing
   or
3. Something added

'Something 'damaged'?

Option one seemed at first to be the favourite. However, I considered it an unlikely candidate, for the simple reason that the food allergic can feel absolutely fine once the reaction wears off. If there was damage at the site, why does it merely last an hour or so during a reaction? One might suggest that the damage is there and that the mere irritation brought about by the incoming allergens is responsible for inflammation which produces the symptoms, and that the inflammation calms down after the hour. But from severe symptoms to complete absence within an hour? I don't think damage perfectly fits the food allergic's picture.

And if 'damage' truly were the cause, my longish experiences of fasting (for two occasions of a month and another of 3 weeks) should have taken care of it by providing freedom from irritation through abstinence. Fasting accelerates healing because of the lack of interference by incoming foodstuffs, so it seems eminently likely that these periods of 'negative nutrition' might have achieved the healing of such 'damage'. But no such healing occurred.

Fasting achieves much healing not only by the absence of often-harmful incoming foods, but because of the certain physiological rest for the entire organism provided by such unburdening of the system. No longer are the body's energies doomed to their usual thankless task of pushing piles of junk foods through 30 feet of tubing. Such wonderful, natural energies can now be fully diverted to another natural mechanism – repair (healing). And that is why many recoveries from all manner of symptoms occur during long therapeutic fasts.

For damage to persist for 30 years, all the time repairing itself within the hour after each allergic reaction, and for it consistently to return when it meets its next meal? That seemed unlikely to say the least. I therefore put something damaged in the 'unlikely candidate' category.

Something 'missing'?

The second option, something missing, also seemed doomed. As I had personally persevered with the all-natural diet for seven full months, I would have thought that if anything were missing in the way of nutrients or other elements, such an intensive natural dietary regimen would, in that time, have corrected it. Often, if a person is ill with a nutrient deficiency, the more severely deficient he is, the quicker he will respond to improved nutritional management.

Besides, if something was 'missing' at the site of the symptom, why was it missing only for the hour or so of the allergic reaction? The something missing hypothesis had also to be put on the back burner.

Something 'added'?

Everything pointed, therefore, to something added being the main factor involved in the food allergy reaction.

Most illness is due to toxaemia - poisoning of the system - according to the doctrine of Nature Cure. Taking patients off harmful diets and returning them to safe natural ones often results in recovered health. It would certainly seem a harmless and reasonable approach to health disorders. Improving your eating habits to approximately those intended by Nature can only be good for you.

So, could the something added be a chemical from past dietary indiscretions, or indeed a drug, lodged within the system? If my something added was just such a toxic substance then why didn't the fast, which is the most efficacious eliminator of all, achieve its removal? And why didn't my seven months on the Gerson therapy (slow but effective) achieve the desired elimination of toxins, if that was indeed the problem? I excluded many of the possible suspect substances such as old drug or chemical deposits, as my previous therapies should have dislodged them.

The drug possibility, my favoured option, was eventually discarded in the something added category. Fasting and the Gerson therapy have been famous for the elimination of drugs (cancer patients have been known to eliminate chemotherapeutic agents from their system whilst on the diet). Yet my recovery from food allergies did not take place whilst fasting or on the Gerson.

I also favoured chemicals, either inhaled from the environment or consumed in processed foods. Perfumes, toothpaste, and many other chemicals to which we are exposed, were weighed up. But again, if drugs or old chemicals in the system were responsible for the food allergy reaction, why should they only cause problems for an hour or so, when they must surely be present permanently?

The drug theory made no sense of why my symptoms - and those of many other food allergics - disappeared entirely when we had a fever.

Another reason I dismissed drugs is that any residues not eliminated would be stored in the adipose tissues of the body. They would not be freely involved with blood flow. They would be 'hidden' to all intents and purposes from the main flow of blood. I shall have more to say about blood flow later on.

By eliminating the 'something damaged' and the 'something missing' as the primary causes of food allergy, we were left with 'something added' as the main offender. But if it wasn't a 'toxic substance', an old drug or chemical, what was it?

Blood flow during allergic reactions

I had long speculated that if the symptom appears repeatedly at one site in the body, then there could be blood flow interference at that site. After all, if there were a rich supply of blood to the problem area then surely that part of the body would be bathed in sufficient nutrients, blood, and oxygen to ensure healthy functioning. I suggest that, in a food allergic 'reaction', the rich supply of blood is being denied or restricted in its access for some reason.

I investigated my reduced blood flow theory by approaching the Royal Infirmary of Edinburgh requesting they use the most up-to-date equipment (Doppler MRI) on me, twice; once when I was relatively symptom-free, and then an hour or so later after consuming an allergic drink of organic juice. The fuller story of the blood flow investigation appears in the next chapter.

Getting back to the something added hypothesis, if the blood flow was normal before the arrival of the incoming allergenic food, then one could reasonably deduce that the something added within the body at the site of the symptom was changing shape or activity, in order to produce interference with the blood flow to that area, if such altered blood flow was at the root of food allergic reactions.

Working on the assumption that there was a blood flow disturbance at the site of the symptom, it seemed unlikely that an inert substance such as a toxin could change shape in order to achieve blockage, merely upon exposure to some incoming allergenic substance, especially when one remembers that even inhalation can produce a reaction.

Most food allergics react to specific substances, repeatedly. Which means that if there is something added, then whatever it is has a special affinity with specific incoming allergens, over and over again.

If there is changed blood flow, it occurs only when particular, specific, substances enter the body. The something added must be changing shape or activity when 'it' recognises the specific incoming allergens with which it has an affinity, and doesn't change shape when other substances are consumed. What then could be changing shape? As I had already ruled out damage, and in that I included inflammation which might account for the changing shape (swelling), as any such damage would most likely have healed during the many periods of fasting, I was left with one highly unusual possibility.

Could the something added be living? That is, could it be a parasite? Could there be a nest of parasites at the site of the symptom? That would certainly give a reasonable explanation for several things, not least the special, selective, affinity this 'something added' had for specific substances. It would also give a reasonable explanation for the changing shape or activity that surely must occur at the problem site during a reaction if there was an altered blood flow at the site.

We examine the parasite possibility shortly, but let us first look at the potential blood flow interference.

5.

Food Allergies and Blood Flow

It was examining the list of complaints of one particular patient that led me to think that perhaps there was a blood flow problem at the site of the symptom, or symptoms, in the food allergic patient.

Martin was a 47 year old who had suffered from vague symptoms for many years. After the usual merry-go-round of doctors and psychiatrists, he eventually latched on to the fact that his symptoms tied in with his eating – and smoking.

I asked him to list all his symptoms when he had his reactions. They were:

1. the face muscles 'pulling down' (very much worse when reacting)
2. poor eyesight
3. poor hearing off and on
4. lots of mouth ulcers
5. receding gums
6. poor skin on scalp
7. poor skin on forehead/nose
8. irritability (much worse when reacting)
9. poor concentration (much worse when reacting)
10. unclear thinking (much worse when reacting)
11. blocked nose
12. chronic tickle in throat
13. much clearing of throat
14. occasional tinnitus
15. poor short term memory (much worse when reacting)

On studying the list, it gradually dawned on me that all these symptoms were in the head area. After confirming with him that he had no mercury fillings or that there could be no dental work which was causing him problems, I came to the conclusion that there had to be a blood flow problem. If that were the case, I thought, could there be a blood flow problem in all food allergics?

Doctors and vascular surgeons I had spoken to on an informal basis had assured me that they had never heard of a connection between diet and blood flow. But long experience told me to carry on looking. After all, as most doctors are not even aware that the food allergy condition exists in the first place, experience told me that they could still be wrong and my theory could indeed be right.

The food allergy syndrome had long been dismissed by orthodox medicine, if for no other reason than that a whole range of seemingly unconnected disorders was linked to it. The sheer number of symptoms associated with food allergy reduces the credibility of the syndrome in their eyes. However, as I knew full well that patients like Martin, and indeed myself, suffered severely on eating apparently ordinary foods, the condition unquestionably existed.

Deciding to find out one way or another whether there could be a blood flow interference, I approached a vascular surgeon privately with my theory. I could only test it if I enlisted the help of orthodox medicine.

It was no surprise to receive the reaction that he didn't 'believe' in the food allergy condition at all, but he listened to what I had to say. I explained how I was convinced there was a blood flow connection and that as a food allergic individual, I wanted to progress matters further by testing with the most up-to-date means available. He was clearly very interested but didn't think there was the slightest chance that what I was proposing would be confirmed. I suggested I wanted a blood flow test done, twice: the first one to be carried out before consuming an allergenic dietary substance and the second, an hour or so later, after consuming the food. He was intrigued at my request and, much to his credit, arranged the tests for me at the Royal Infirmary of Edinburgh, with a colleague of his who was a 'highly experienced radiologist'.

While I knew that the testing would be by Doppler equipment – used in hospitals throughout the world – I was fearful that any hypoperfusion, if it existed, might be in the smaller arterioles and so not be picked up. Only by the SPECT (single photon emission tomographic) method could any interference in blood flow in the microcirculation be picked up, and I didn't particularly want to go down that road as it was invasive, whereas the Doppler was not.

When the day came to be tested at the Royal Infirmary I was, thankfully, pretty symptom free. The entire exercise would have been useless if I had been feeling unwell to start with, as reduced blood flow would exist from the very outset if my theory were correct.

However, I went fully prepared for the test not to show up anything of real value, as I really felt that any changes would be in the undetectable microcirculation. I took with me to the hospital a flask containing organic carrot and cabbage juice, to which I knew I was allergic.

I had an animated conversation with the doctor who was conducting the testing, about what the likely outcome would be. He knew, as did his vascular surgeon friend, of 'food allergies', but he too was apprehensive of their existence and their supposed mimicking of so many claimed symptoms. He expressed his view – which I thought astonishing – that diet had no part to play in vascular integrity. When I told him I knew of patients who had shown a 'clearing up' of a degree of atherosclerosis after being on a natural diet for some time, he reluctantly admitted that he too knew of similar cases and only said that he didn't believe in it to 'promote conversation'!

He admitted that he had seen a difference in patients with atherosclerosis who, after adhering to a low-cholesterol diet, showed an improved reading on the Doppler test when re-tested at a later date.

I lay on the examination table whilst he greased my carotid artery prior to the test. We freely talked as he was using the ultrasound equipment and watching the results on the monitor in front of him. All looked well and he declared that the carotids were showing good elasticity and that I had nothing to worry about. I had told him what I was going to do – drink my allergenic drink – and that he was to test me again in about an hour. I am sure that he thought he was simply humouring me at such a seemingly bizarre request, but he agreed to do it.

Now, at this stage, I wish to point out that I am not the sort of person who can simply, by mere mental suggestion, influence my blood flow! I am not the susceptible person who, expecting something to happen, will 'suggest' that it happen. If anything, I am so stubborn in my nature that I would probably induce the opposite result. Besides, I truly did not think that the Doppler would be precise enough to give me the result I considered likely; it would almost certainly take the fine tuning of the SPECT to identify any changes.

I put on my shirt whilst he went off to attend to other duties. He said he would be back in about 'half an hour' after I had taken my juices. I would have far preferred a full hour, as experience told me that that was when I would most likely be at the peak of any reaction. But I knew that, as he was a busy doctor, it was difficult for me to dictate to him what to do. Besides, I thought nothing would show, and, as a firm non-believer, he definitely thought it would be a waste of time!

After about half an hour, the doctor returned. I told him that I wasn't fully reacting, but that I felt 'something'; hopefully enough to register some kind of response. I was trying to suggest he come back in about another half hour, but how I could say that without appearing dictatorial was beyond me, so I just had to get on with it.

It was clear he had used the Doppler equipment many, many, times before and was thoroughly familiar with the readings that would be produced. The combination of my not getting the full hour that I wanted and the manner in which he showed total confidence that there would be no change in the readings both served somewhat to demoralise me.

I was now convinced that, after several years harbouring this theory, now that I finally had the equipment at my disposal, it was going to give no meaningful result at all. My theory, plausible though it might have been, was now going to die an ignominious death.

The conversation picked up and animated chit-chat took over as he confidently applied the probe to my carotids again, whilst watching the pulsating images on the screen in front of him.

All of a sudden he stopped the conversation in its tracks and, quickly putting his finger to his lips, said 'Shhhh'. He was avidly studying the screen and obviously trying to make sense of what he was seeing. Much to his horror, the Doppler ultrasound equipment WAS registering a significant change in blood flow perfusion!

He was moving the probe over the carotids again and again to see if the reading would alter. But it wouldn't. There was no disputing that this second reading showed a significant change in blood flow from the first.

According to John Buckley, Director of the Arterial Disease Clinic in Leigh, near Manchester, Doppler ultrasound equipment is accurate to plus or minus five percent. My reading at the Royal Infirmary of Edinburgh showed a *thirty percent* change on the second reading, indicative of a considerably reduced blood flow!

Somewhat irritated that someone not in his 'field' of expertise could predict such an unlikely result right in front of him, he could only bluster out 'but it's not scientific!'. Yes, I agreed with him. It wasn't scientific. But it was half way there. All it needed was more tests on more people. Just because this test does not have the luxury of other tests to compare it with, does not mean to say it won't prove to be valid when, eventually, scientifically approved testing is carried out. Every 'discovery', no matter how important, starts with a first test which can't be corroborated until the next tests are carried out.

Besides, if he were truly a man of science, instead of dismissing what could have been an important finding, he should have initiated a full-scale investigation and trials, to see if simple eating truly could influence, every time, blood flow in patients who were so predisposed.

If he were truly seeking to help his many patients, he should have swallowed his pride, taken on board this unlikely finding and pursued it to a conclusion, to determine whether or not it was repeatable. He should have ascertained its validity by further tests, instead of dismissing it simply because he was professionally embarrassed that someone 'unskilled' in his discipline could add a new dimension to what he very likely considered his unsurpassed skills in radiology. He should have considered even more carefully that it might not be a freak result because of the fact that this unusual finding was *predicted in advance*.

Regardless, as the change of reading came as a result of consuming an allergen, all indicators pointed to that allergen being responsible. I had not exercised. I had not climbed stairs. I had not left the small room. I had not eaten that morning. No early morning breakfast could have been responsible – only the carrot/cabbage juice consumed in between the two tests.

So, my theory was proven – to me at least! This also finally answers those critics who pooh-pooh the food allergic condition because of the sheer number of disorders associated with it. As every part of the body is supplied with blood, therefore the food allergic condition can cause blood flow interference *at any part of the body*, producing *any* symptom!

I soon realised why he should have been horrified, why he should have been so reluctant to accept the findings as shown. If it really was the case that ordinary foods could so dramatically influence the readings on the Doppler, and if it really was the case that food 'allergies' were so truly widespread, then it would throw all or any of his future testings into serious doubt.

From now on in, he could never be sure if Joe Bloggs whom he might test next had just eaten his allergenic breakfast and that the reading he was now seeing was not a true one but a 'post-allergen' reading! All manner of doubt might now creep into the picture with virtually ANY of the patients who come to be tested. Notwithstanding, I was happy with the result and decided to investigate this further.

I knew that Attention Deficit Hyperactivity Disorder (ADHD) children were, in reality, food allergy victims. I also knew that studies carried out by Prof. Hans Lou in Denmark, involving nine school-age ADHD sufferers showed a reduced striatal blood flow.[2] The mean flow was 10.7ml/100g/min lower than the mean of the control group of 15 age-and-sex-matched children. Furthermore, flow to the thalamic regions was also reduced significantly (by 7.3ml/100g/min).

This study did not look at, or even consider, a food involvement; I merely introduce this ADHD study as evidence of cerebral blood flow involvement in a condition that has a known food-allergen connection.

The hyperactive-child link to food/chemical/environmental allergens will be known to most readers familiar with food allergy. Returning to the blood flow link to food allergies, separately, and not at all connected, there have been studies that show migraines have a blood flow involvement and others that have shown that migraines could be brought on by eating allergenic foods.

Now, these studies have not been linked. The one showing a blood flow involvement never considered a dietary connection but merely showed the sufferer had a hypoperfusion. The other studies showing diet is involved in migraines considered not for one moment a blood flow involvement. However simple the leap from one to the other should have been, it hadn't been made. No studies showing that migraine can be brought on by consuming an allergenic substance AND that there is a concomitant blood flow hypoperfusion, have thus far been made.

There was one study in Japan that came near it and is an example of how a before-and-after case of blood flow interference linked to diet allergy could have been missed but was simply not considered or suspected. Carried out in 1994 at the Toyama University Hospital in Japan, the study showed that cerebral ischaemia in a 33-year-old woman migraine sufferer was reversible.[3] Using the SPECT images, they discovered cerebral ischaemia during the migraine attack but when tested when she was symptom-free, no such ischaemia existed!

As we know full well that migraine is a classic food-allergy-related disorder, the study missed that one final bit to round off the three-way connection between blood flow, diet, and symptoms: it didn't address the issue of what the lady was allergic to in the first place to produce the migraine. Had it done so, the three-way connection could have been made.

One Italian study confirmed a food intolerance in ALL of the 43 paediatric patients with migraine under study.[4] Again, however, no blood flow consideration was made. Thomsen, Iversen and Olesen of the University of Copenhagen confirmed, in 1995 that cerebral blood flow velocities are reduced during attacks of migraine.[5] Elsewhere, fifteen patients with migraine displayed reduced blood flow when tested in Denmark in 1993.[6]

There are other medical 'similarities'. Whilst the three-way connection is never made, there are many conditions that produce inflammation of a blood vessel in any one particular place in the body which then produces reduced blood flow.

The diagnostic label then given will only be to the visible presenting symptom. That is, a migraine-type headache will be diagnosed 'migraine'. It will not be labelled as 'pronounced headache due to cerebral hypoperfusion'.

Reduced blood flow due to temporarily inflamed blood vessels elsewhere in the body will similarly be given the name of the condition obvious to the physician examining the patient at that time. The arthritic patient may well have a food-allergy connection but simply present with arthritis in the knee. The doctor will diagnose it as simply arthritis. But further investigation would find that (i) there is a dietary involvement, and (ii) there is a blood flow interference. However, commonly both (i) and (ii) are missed.

Hypersensitivity vasculitis is a recognised condition involving blood vessel inflammation and hence, hypoperfusion. Looking through the published medical literature, a 1992 study showed 5 patients with hypersensitivity vasculitis were put on an elimination diet in order to see if food could be responsible for the condition.[7] Four patients achieved a complete remission and one patient experienced great improvement on the elimination diet. In three cases the vasculitis relapsed following the introduction of food additives; in one case with the addition of potatoes and green vegetables (beans and green peas) and in the last case with the addition of eggs to the diet. The offending foods and additives were subsequently eliminated from the usual diet and no relapses were observed in two years of follow-up.

It was in 1866 that Kussmaul and Maier first accurately described an inflammatory disease of the medium-sized and small arteries and named that condition periarteritis nodosa, also known as PAN. Whilst they recognised that these larger blood vessels could as be affected by such inflammation, they also recognised that the small arterioles and even veins can be similarly affected. Juergens *Peripheral Vascular Diseases* adds: 'Despite the advances in modern medicine however, little can be added today to what Kussmaul and Maier described and reported more than a century ago'.

PAN can be involved in blood flow interference by virtue of inflamed arteries, and such blood flow interference can involve virtually any part of the body. The most common sites are the heart, kidneys, alimentary tract, liver, pancreas and nervous system. Ross and Wilson's *Anatomy and Physiology* further states that PAN is 'usually acute at first but may become chronic. . . . It is believed to be caused by an immune reaction'.

In 1942, Arnold Rice Rich, a Professor of Pathology from Alabama, did a study on the relationship between periarteritis nodosa and hypersensitivity. He published his clinical observations on 'The Role of Hypersensitivity in Periarteritis Nodosa'. He studied seven patients with pneumonia or meningitis in whom PAN developed whilst they were receiving antiserum and (in most cases) sulphonamide therapy. He concluded that 'These cases. . . indicate that vascular lesions of this type can be a manifestation of the anaphylactic type of hypersensitivity, and suggest the importance of a search for the inciting antigen in cases of periarteritis nodosa that come under clinical observation'.

It is abundantly clear that (i) many seemingly 'unconnected' symptoms are indeed linked to dietary/chemical/environmental-allergen influence, and (ii) the offending dietary/chemical/environmental-allergen can produce interference in blood flow, and (iii) the three-way connection between symptom, allergen, and blood flow, is virtually never recognised or considered.

6.

Enter the Human Parasite!

In a Gerson Therapy newsletter as far back as 1992 I had postulated the theory that there was something 'inert' at the site of the symptom within the food allergic, something that became 'active' when that person consumed – or inhaled – an allergenic substance. The possibility of that 'inert' something being a human parasite did not cross my mind at that time. But it was now becoming a strong candidate for being the 'something added' for which I had been searching.

Many questions answered

If the existence of parasites at the site of the symptom can cause the allergy problem, then many longstanding puzzles about the condition can finally be addressed, among them the question of affinity to specific (allergenic) substances and not to others. Parasites, like any living animal, will have specific nutritional requirements, met by plundering, or sharing, the host's nutrition.

Parasite existence would also explain why food allergic patients often recall that their problem occurred at the time of a death in the family, a divorce, a break-up with a lover, even an injury or other trauma. Parasites are known to invade a body that is under stress; whose defences, if you like, are down.

The hereditary factor attached to 'allergies' could also be explained: parasites can reproduce within the human, enter the man's sperm, pass through intercourse to the mother, then pass via the mother's bloodstream to the offspring.

With some degree of optimism I proceeded to explore the subject of human parasitology. It soon became apparent that parasitology is the step-child of modern medicine. Hardly any medical student chooses the subject for specialisation. It seems generally considered as only applicable to third-world countries and not to be relevant to everyday general practice in our modern, 'sophisticated' world...

Whilst knowledge of human parasitology is ever-evolving, there is clearly much to be learned in its connection to common health disorders. Even the connection between animal parasitism and human health is only now becoming apparent. In *The Biology of Parasitism* (Alan R. Liss Inc. New York) it states: 'There are many infections which were generally thought to be restricted to animals and are now known to be capable of transmission to man'.

If medical science has failed to connect symptoms of disease to something as highly visible and obvious as our food – and it has – then it should be no surprise that the connection between health disorders and virtually invisible organisms such as parasites has passed it by.

Modern-day parasite infestation should not be considered all that unlikely. After all, with high-speed travel and the circumnavigation of the globe within an increasing number of people's reach, parasites can be picked up abroad and transported, within the host and by kind permission of the airlines, back to Great Britain, America, or any other developed country. Parasites can be carried back from holiday. Parasites do not recognise borders or languages; they will go where you go, if you are kind enough to transport them.

One highly possible, if initially improbable scenario relating to my own food allergic illness is that my grandfather, who was a Captain with the Royal Flying Corps during the First World War, and who visited Egypt, India, and other exotic countries, could have picked up parasites there and brought them back to this country. As I now know my grandfather had awful mood swings that seemed eminently capable of being considered food allergic, then I could assume he too was an unwitting sufferer of the condition. We also know there is a strong hereditary factor in the food allergy disorder.

The parasites could then have reproduced, as they can, within his body, and made him their permanent host. He could then have passed the strain to my grandmother, who could in turn have passed it to the foetus that was to become my father. His life was bedevilled by chronic, severe, asthma, then by alcoholism, which he claimed was a result of seeking respite from his breathing difficulties. Apparently the alcohol helped him to breathe more easily.

Mood swings, asthma, even alcoholism all have hereditary tie-ins. They also have strong food allergy implications. In turn, I could have been born with the parasite, inactive or inert within my body until a trauma (a break-up with a girlfriend) brought about the now-recognised condition which became known as my food allergy.

Whilst that parasite journey from my grandfather cannot be proved, neither should it entirely be discounted. There are well over a hundred different kinds of human parasites. They can enter man in his diet, by his eating their virtually-invisible eggs on fruits and other foods, through his skin, through any of the orifices and even by the inhalation of airborne micro-organisms.

They can invade virtually any organ or tissue in the human host. They can be found in the sperm. Such is the mode of transport the HIV-virus pursues and the spread of such a parasite (for that is what it is) is by means of intercourse. During intercourse, this parasite can be transmitted to the mother's body and enter the foetus via the mother's bloodstream. The child can then be born, an unwitting carrier of the parasite, which can lie 'dormant' for many years before something triggers activation, and illness finally appears.

These parasites can live within the host for decades, if not for the host's entire life. The 'trigger' that re-activates the virus can be some weakening of the host's system, often at a time of mental or physical trauma, or injury. Even the trauma involved in an operation in hospital can be the spark for a new illness.

Parasites are known to inhabit their host when it is at its weakest, which fits perfectly with what we know about food allergies. It is almost universally the case that people who develop food allergies do so soon after some trauma in their lives, such as bereavement, divorce, or illness.

One particular parasite found in man – the *schistosome* – has three sub-species: *Schistosoma mansoni*, *haematobium* and *japonicum*. Between them these are currently estimated to affect over 200 million people, mainly in S. America and the Caribbean, Africa and, to a lesser extent, the Near East and China, as well as Southeast Asia and the Philippines. Although a small percentage of sufferers will eventually die from the parasites, many others will suffer more or less severe chronic ill-health. It is the chronic ill health link to these micro-organisms and organisms like them that should concern us.

The *schistosome* life cycle in man can be two to five years. The adult worms seek refuge in the pelvic veins. The eggs can pass up the hepatic portal vein and lodge in the liver or they can pass out through the intestinal wall and into the faeces.

Parasites of man appear to know exactly where to lodge in the human form; they 'migrate' around the body until they settle in their favoured habitat. This migration can cause fleeting symptoms, e.g. itching, in different areas of the body as they pass through.

The parasite possibility

In an attempt to connect my food allergy condition to parasitic activity, I contacted a local hospital and asked for a parasite test. They required a single stool sample, which was then sent to the Liverpool School of Tropical Medicine. Disappointingly, the result came back negative. That meant that I should probably eliminate parasites as being at the root of my food allergy problem. But the more I thought about parasites, the more they seemed an extremely probable scenario.

I decided not to eliminate the possibility entirely, merely to shelve it for the time being, waiting to see if anything in the future would 'bring it back into the picture'. About two years later, I came across a book that was to do just that. I found someone else who had considered parasites as being at the root of much illness; Dr. Hulda Clark of California.

Her books *The Cure for All Diseases* and *The Cure for All Cancers* may appear to have contentious titles, but on examining the contents, I found her theories made eminent sense.

I travel to California

Dr. Clark uses electronic methods to identify human parasites in her patients and she is adamant that most modern illnesses, including all cancers, are the result of parasite infestation.

That cancer should be linked to parasite activity is not new. *Bailliere's Nurses' Dictionary* (21st Edition; 1994) states under Virus: . . . . 'there is evidence that certain viruses may be capable of causing cancer'. And Dr. Roger Wyburn-Mason, a British researcher who wrote *The Causation of Rheumatoid Disease* and *Many Human Cancers: A New Concept in Medicine* was also aware of the link between parasites and cancer and, indeed, between parasites and a classic food allergy condition, rheumatoid arthritis.[8] Dr. Wyburn-Mason pointed to the parasite *Endolimax nana* as being implicated not only in rheumatoid arthritis but in many other illnesses as well.

Couple that knowledge to the many recoveries from both cancer and arthritis by patients on Nature Cure diets like the Gerson, and we notice that there exists a means of eradicating cancer, arthritis, and their parasitic instigators all with the same method – the adopting of a natural diet!

Whilst Dr. Clark appears not to have the dietary knowledge that goes with the Gerson therapy, her approach to parasitic elimination takes a more direct route, by attempting to kill the parasites by herbal means and by use of her electronic 'zapper' equipment.

An independent scientist, Dr. Clark began her studies in biology at the University of Saskatchewan in Canada, where she was awarded the Bachelor of Arts, Magna Cum Laude, and the Master of Arts, with High Honours. After two years of study at McGill University she attended the University of Minnesota studying biophysics and cell physiology, receiving her Doctorate degree in physiology in 1958. She left government funded research in 1979 and began private consulting on a full time basis. It was eleven years after this that she started to notice the clues implicating parasites in cancer.

Whilst the equipment that she uses, a synchrometer, may leave many people querying its efficacy, because it involves identifying and interpreting various ranges of frequencies that all living organisms produce, the science behind it seems entirely sound.

Having travelled to California to see it in use and receive basic training in the approach, I am convinced she has a sound basis for her belief that most illnesses have a parasitic connection. I admire Dr. Clark immensely for taking a major step in the identification of what appears to be a major factor in illness.

Herbs

As stated, Dr. Clark uses herbs and an electronic 'zapper' to kill parasites. But she is aware of their limitations as far as total eradication of the problem is concerned. In line with the advice of clinical ecologists, she recommends the elimination from your home environment of most household chemicals and other pollutants. When I visited San Diego, I was privileged to meet Carmen Myers, an assistant to Dr. Clark, and an expert in the use of the synchrometer. She taught me and other class members the rudiments of the technique. Carmen was able to identify several parasites and undesirable bacteria in me. The parasites found in my body were:

Ascaris; Strongyloides; Fasciola hepatica.

Among the many smaller micro-organisms (bacteria) found in my body were;

Mycobacterium phlei;
Clostridium botulinum;
Clostridium perfringens;
Staphylococcus aureus and *Ergot sclerotium.*

The parasite as the 'something added' in food allergic reactions was well and truly back in the picture.

The *Ascaris* parasite, known to cause asthma in laboratory workers studying this organism, can produce vast numbers of eggs/worms per day.[9] It is estimated that up to 250,000 *Ascaris* offspring can be produced in a single day!

I have already shown that there is blood flow interference during the allergic reaction. This could be a simple blockage of the lumen of the blood vessel, or even air passage, by parasite presence. This hypothesis is strongly borne out by the following quote from *Human Parsitology*: 'This [*Ascaris Pneumonitis*] results from ruptured capillaries during larval passage into the alveoli, or from small infarcts due to blockage of arterioles.'[10]

In other words, the presence of the parasite *Ascaris* in a hollow (or filled) tube such as an artery or alveslus (air passage) can create a simple blockage which results either in blood flow reduction or airflow reduction. Do not the well known allergic conditions of migraine and asthma fit perfectly into such a picture, involving as they do the impeding of both blood flow and air flow respectively?

But why did the test on my stool sample show negative? When I returned to the U.K. I contacted the Liverpool School of Tropical Medicine and was given the answer. They agreed that I could well have parasites. There are many reasons why a single stool sample can show negative. Apparently, no one single sample can act as a true test. Several samples over several days are required and even then there is no guarantee, as not all parasites' eggs appear in every stool sample.

The usual method employed is to look for cysts, trophozoites, ova, eggs or worm segments in random stool samples. There are several reasons why this practice can fail to identify parasitic existence. Parasites can reside in the blood, blood vessel walls, other organs and tissues and will not exist in stool samples. Common childhood parasites like pinworm and dogworms are also rarely seen in stools, as are their eggs. Other parasites cannot be seen in the stool because they live in the gastrointestinal tract lining. They are capable of adhering vice-like to the intestinal mucosa and, unless they are wrenched from their habitat they will not be seen in stool samples.

Further parasite species, such as *strongyloides* and *giardia* for example, have an erratic excretion pattern and this can vary greatly from day to day. Many parasitologists recommend the examination of three to six stool samples, taken on different days. Even these stool samples can be negative whilst all the time the patient plays host to nests of parasites.[11]

Since my investigations into parasites started, I have learned how to microscopically examine my own stool samples for parasites, and it is a wonder to behold when one can actually retrieve such a living organism from your body and yet be almost entirely in the dark as to what extent it may be responsible for your illness. The lifestyle of many parasites is still a mystery and there is much waiting to be learned about their nutritional and physiological requirements, as well as their behaviour within the human organism. At least I now recognised that I *had* parasites and that I *had* food allergies, and that the two were almost certainly linked!

The hidden epidemic

Human parasites have probably been on Earth for as long as man. It is becoming clear that every nation in the world have their own varieties of parasites, just as they have their own species of animal, plant etc. It is also clear that it is not a problem specific to third-world countries, but stretching much further.

I suggest that a great deal of human misery through the centuries has been the direct result of this hidden and unsuspected epidemic. It might well be proven one day that the vast majority of illness is a result of the invasion of micro-organisms, and that this may have been so since time began. After all, if it can be so under-considered even now, in the 21st century, with all the advanced medical and scientific equipment at our disposal, what chance had earlier physicians of making the connection between presenting symptoms and something invisible to the human eye?

It was only with the invention of the microscope that parasitic organisms could be actually seen for the very first time. In 1671, Kircher observed tiny worms in the blood of patients with plague and claimed the worms were responsible for the illness.[12]

However it is likely that what he was viewing were clusters of red blood cells and the true honour of being the first observer of parasitic micro-organisms probably falls to Anthony Leeuwenhoek, a linen-draper from Delft in Holland. Leeuwenhoek's hobby was experimentation with the making of relatively simple microscopes and it was in 1674 that he observed microscopic living animals in rain, pond and sea water as well as various other fluids. He wrote of his observations in a series of letters to the Royal Society in London but it appears neither he nor the Royal Society at that time recognised the significance of his findings.

During the eighteenth century several scientists suggested that the tiny organisms Leeuwenhoek had discovered might be responsible for various diseases, but there was little substantiation of the theory, and it was disregarded.

By the early 19th century advances in microscope design had made possible the description and categorisation of some of these micro-organisms. In 1838 Ehrenberg, in his work on Infusoria (the small creatures found in infusions), introduced such terms as bacterium, vibrio, spirillum and spirochaete. In 1835, Agostino Bassi had described the fungus which caused muscardine, a disease of silkworms, and he had suggested that this disease was transmitted by contact or by infection of food. This, the first reliable report of a disease caused by a transmissible parasitic micro-organism, was followed in 1839 by Schoenlein's description of the fungus that causes the human disease favus.

In 1850 Rayer and Davaine reported the presence of rod-shaped organisms in the blood of animals that had died of anthrax, and Davaine later showed that this disease could be transmitted by inoculation of blood containing such rods, but not of blood from which they were absent.

Mental illness

Mental illness related to food allergy is extremely common. Or, to put it another way, it is extremely common to find a food link to mental symptoms.

Depression is probably the most frequent complaint made by sufferers of food allergy. Other 'psychiatric' symptoms have been shown to be influenced by incoming foodstuffs and it is often suggested by those practitioners knowledgeable of the mental connection in food allergy, that psychiatric wards up and down the country might be emptied virtually overnight were proper food-allergy investigations to be carried out on these patients.

So too with prisons. Food allergy problems are almost certainly the reason behind much criminal, even violent, activity. Indeed, the link between diet and teenage delinquency was the subject of a BBC Television programme entitled *Little Monsters*, transmitted on 29th April 1992. This showed a 'miraculous' change in a group of problem children's violent behaviour when the culprit foodstuffs were eliminated from their diets, only for the unacceptable behaviour to quickly return on the re-introduction of the offending foods.

The connection between food allergies and the children's criminal behaviour was so clear-cut, so striking, that the West Yorkshire Superintendent of police hit the headlines at the time when he went public with his statement that a juvenile delinquent had given up a life of crime after he'd been discovered to be allergic to milk and tomatoes!

Remember too, that the link between mental disorders, criminal activity and unacceptable behaviour, does not simply apply to 'juveniles'. The unacceptable behaviour does not suddenly stop when the child reaches voting age. It will continue as long as that person is unaware of the link between his eating habits and his criminal behaviour – as will be the case in the majority of all prisoners. There surely exists a massive number of adult delinquents.

If blood flow in the brain is disturbed during food allergy reactions, it should be no surprise that mental symptoms, and indeed criminal activity, might result from such cerebral malfunction.

As we are now linking parasitic activity to food allergy disorder, and as parasites seek out specific habitats within the host to infest - the brain being a common site for such habitation – then it should be no surprise that adverse, or distortion of, mental function can result.

On their migration through the body to their desired organ or tissues, parasitic micro-organisms can settle in the brain, adhering to blood vessel walls, causing all manner of thought process distortion to occur when the blood flow is interrupted.

The bizarre thought processes that are the lot of the schizophrenic may well be due to the presence of micro-organisms residing at the part of the brain that controls these particular emotions.

Nervous system invasion by viruses can follow various routes. Some blood-borne viruses localize in cerebral vessels and invade adjacent brain tissue, whereas others penetrate the capillaries of the blood-CSF junction in the meninges or the choroid plexus. Remember also that viruses are also parasites.

Origins

The word 'parasite' comes from the Greek words *para* which means beside and *sitos* meaning food. There are two distinct types of parasites: those that live inside the body, called endoparasites, and those that live on the outside of the body, called ectoparasites. The animal or human that becomes infected is referred to as the 'host'.

The majority of parasites do not kill their host, but use him or her either as an intermediate stage in their development, at the end of which they will move out and seek another organism to inhabit, or as a permanent home within that host for the entire duration of their lifecycle. They will reproduce within the host, resulting in the human becoming the unwitting host to these lodgers for his entire lifespan. Whilst most parasites will 'only' make the host feel unwell, either physically or mentally, some, known as parasitoids, eventually kill their host.

Parasites vary in size, from worms several feet long which can live in your intestines, to smaller worms, medium-sized amoebae, bacteria, and, the smallest of all, viruses. The worms themselves can be microscopically small or as thin as hairs.

Parasites have their own preferred sites, or organs, in the bodies of their target hosts. They might enter the host through the skin, or be swallowed inadvertently as microscopically-small eggs on foodstuffs. Once in the system they will proceed to travel through the body, seeking out their desired organ or tissue in which to live. Undoubtedly the conditions at the chosen site have to be perfect for the propagation of the parasite species and it will be these specific conditions peculiar to each parasite that will determine the specificity of the host's target organs or tissues.

Arthritis

Because they do not have a skeletal structure, parasites do not show up on X-rays. It is for that very reason that the likely widespread existence of human parasites is entirely unsuspected. It would take a most unusual doctor to suddenly consider that the arthritic patient he has been dealing with for years, with all the classic symptoms of the condition, might have the illness because of parasitic presence at the site in the body where the arthritis is. Having established the patient's condition years ago as being arthritis, that generally is all he needs to know, and his future management of that patient's condition will be with medication.

However, the condition of arthritis is a well-known one in food allergy circles; it has long been known amongst Clinical Ecologists that there inevitably *is* a food link to the disorder.

We can now suggest, with a fair degree of confidence, that micro-organism presence will indeed be at the site of the symptom. Furthermore, as we now know that there is a blood flow interference at the site of the symptom, then we can then point to the allergic patient with arthritis and state that;

(i) Yes, his condition is arthritic.

(ii) The arthritis will flare up with foods or drinks; that is, the patient's condition will be labelled 'food allergic'.

(iii) There will be almost certainly a blood flow interference at the site of the symptom.

(iv) There will almost certainly be parasitic micro-organisms at the site of the symptom.

But can we be sure that the condition well-known as arthritis, truly is caused by invading micro-organisms? At least one outbreak of arthritis has indeed been shown to be caused by an invading micro-organism.

Lyme Disease is a condition that was first 'discovered' in Lyme, Connecticut, USA.[13] It first appeared in epidemic form in 1975, when some 51 residents of several communities around the Connecticut village of Old Lyme developed rheumatoid arthritis. Unusually, it was specially rife amongst the younger residents. It was probably because of the unusually young age of the sufferers that further investigation was undertaken. That investigation turned up parasites as being the main player in the condition! Whilst all the symptoms presented were identical to arthritis, the cause of the condition turned out to be ticks – tiny mites that normally feed on animals but which can transfer to humans.

The ticks carried a germ – a parasitic bacterium called *borrelia* or *rickettsia* – which migrated to the joints and caused the inflammation that produced the symptoms of arthritis. It wasn't long before sufferers of arthritis in Britain began to show the parasite in blood tests when examined.

That any symptom of an arthritic nature has been shown to be of parasitic origin makes it vital to do further research to see if other, perhaps *all* arthritises can be the result of parasitic infestation. And if the common symptom of arthritis can be so parasitically linked, and as arthritis is an extremely common food allergy complaint, what price all symptoms of food allergy now being linked to parasities?

A study in America in 1995 carried out by P.W. Paparone on a patient with hypothyroidism (a condition linked to low body temperature) concurrent with Lyme Disease, concluded:

> Lyme disease can be seen as localized, disseminated, acute, or chronic and can mimic other, more serious diseases. Even though it is a multisystemic illness, very few spirochetes (parasites) are present; yet once established in the host, it can persist for many years. The antibody response is slow and variable and the spirochete is difficult to isolate from clinical specimens, even those obtained from the pathognomonic skin lesion.[14]

These variables, together with non-specific symptoms, make the diagnosis of Lyme disease very difficult. Paparone concluded that the diagnosis of Lyme disease could 'easily have been missed' because of the hypothyroidism present. It may be that the vast majority of patients presenting to their doctor with 'arthritis' will have parisitic infestation at the site of the symptoms, something which may never even have entered the doctor's head.

After it was discovered in the USA, Lyme disease raised its head everywhere, including Britain, where many cases were reported. They had of course existed all along, but no-one had identified them as of parasitic origin.

This phenomenon is not uncommon in medicine. Once something has been identified, then more clinicians begin to look for it, and lo and behold, it appears here, there and everywhere. *Helicobacter pylorus*, the parasite linked to duodenal ulcers, was initially dismissed by science, but is now commonly identified and accepted. Common sense suggests that the parasite will have existed within these patients' bodies all along.

Dr. Hulda Clark is not the only researcher who has observed the link between a host of common illnesses, including cancers, and parasitic presence within the patient. Recent research by Prof. Jan Walboomers of the Free University in Amsterdam, has linked a parasite – the HPV virus – to 99.7% of cervical cancers. This is the first time that scientists have been able to identify with such confidence a specific parasite for any human cancer. The finding that parasites can be involved in cancer at all is perhaps a first step towards identifying the involvement of many other such organisms in many more illnesses.

Ann Louise Gittleman, in her book *Guess What Came to Dinner,* states that 'massive food and environmental allergies have all been reported when amoebas are found in the system'. Here again we have further evidence that there is some connection between food allergies and parasites.

If, as suggested, approximately 80% of all patients who present to their doctor with health problems have hidden food allergies, and if parasitic infestation at the site of the symptom is the cause of such disorders, then we are truly talking about parasitic infestation of epidemic proportions!

However, recognising that your health problem exists because of parasite activity within your body, is one thing, eliminating it is quite another. Let us now address that issue.

7.

How to Eliminate Parasites

I decided to try Dr. Clark's parasite killing programme of herbs to see if it would have any influence on my food allergy condition. I have tried hundreds of cure-alls in my time and a host of nutritional supplements, all claiming to cure the allergy condition. Not one has worked. None has even remotely been near removing my ever-present symptoms.

I can report that, within 2 days of taking the herbs, my symptoms were reduced dramatically! However they returned two days later. Perhaps I had taken the adult parasites 'by surprise' and the offspring, emerging from their protected larval stage, took over the work of their parents – who knows, but the possibility must be considered. I am not the sort of person to fall prey to suggestion, especially after my failures with many earlier supplements or therapies. I had taken the parasite herbs with my normal degree of scepticism.

The fact that they cleared my symptoms at all was a major breakthrough. True, it lasted only a short time, but one must never lose sight of the fact that, even if for only a day or two, it was the first product in over 30 years to do so.

It further confirmed to me that there must be some parasitic involvement in my condition. Though disappointed that the improvement didn't last, I was nevertheless encouraged to feel I was on the right track.

The acknowledged and accepted practice to eliminate any parasite is to attempt to kill it directly. Dr. Clark utilises herbal parasiticides for this purpose. But the mere taking of such herbal preparations does not guarantee complete recovery. She, as well as some German Nature Cure specialists – Heilpraktikers – who are now looking into the subject, recognises that parasites invariably re-infest the patient after apparently being killed. Other steps have to be taken, for example, boiling dairy products to eliminate such parasites and bacteria. Dr. Clark also recommends having a 'dental clean-up' which can mean not only the removal of all mercury, but a considerable overhaul of the entire dentistry in the mouth, including the removal of teeth which have had root canal work carried out on them. Unfortunately, even after removal, patients would very often still have symptoms.

Killing the parasites is not the full solution to the problem. It should be recognised that parasites go through many stages; they can live 40 years or more in a human and reproduce all that time. They often die only when the patient dies! An indication of their apparent indestructibility is the fact that bacteria, *three million years old*, were resuscitated after lying all that time dormant in Siberian permafrost!

Whilst the parasiticidal herbs may kill or immobilise the adult parasites, the larvae can survive unscathed and continue their parents' work once they hatch, starting the problem all over again. That's what I meant by taking the 'parents' by surprise! There had to be another way to eliminate parasites, other than merely swallowing a substance in an attempt to kill them, especially when the results do not last.

The amount of care that Dr. Clark – understandably – advises in an attempt to avoid all contact with parasites, is huge. Virtually all dairy products have to be boiled before eating, and all fruits and vegetables have to be thoroughly scrubbed and washed. Dr. Clark advises careful removal of all dirt from vegetables, so that no parasite eggs may be consumed. She recommends sterilising your toothbrush with grain alcohol each time you use it as well as many other suggestions such as not licking your fingers when turning over the pages of a book.

But, as hygienically sound as this approach may appear, one wonders how it is that people who *do* lick their fingers when turning over pages can remain free from illness. There is perhaps a limit to the avoidance measures one can take. No animal in nature washes its food before consuming it.

I have seen, as we probably all have, television documentaries showing tigers and lions eating their kill raw. I have watched to see if they take in dirt in the process, and they all do. They do not have the facilities to wash and clean the carcass; dirt is part and parcel of their 'diet'. Yet they are healthy and powerful beasts. It is only modern man who suffers all manner of maladies.

I could only conclude that Dr. Clark's well-meaning but highly clinical approach to eating is not the right way to look at the problem. No one wants to eat dirt, so we would normally clean the produce anyway, but as parasite eggs are microscopic, some would inevitably enter the average person's body. Yet not everyone becomes ill. There had to be more to the parasite problem than attempting to avoid all contact with them, an impossibility in any case.

Parasites are all around us!

To give you some insight into the ubiquitous nature of unwanted creatures in or on our food, let me quote from a recent newspaper article:

Mites – teeny spidery jobs – are infiltrating our food, a conference was told this week. They multiply like crazy in grain stores, getting into our flour, bread and breakfast bowls. One baby cereal tested contained over 20,000 mites per kilo. And they're not all dead either.[15]

In truth, it's almost impossible to ensure food is totally animal free. In America, there are government guidelines on how much 'animal extras' are permissable. That's right – how MUCH. For instance, two rodent hairs per pound of popcorn, three fly eggs per ounce of tomato juice, five maggots per ounce of canned mushrooms and one percent of mammal excreta in peppercorns.

A sampling of 6 types of vegetable in an American study[16] which was carried out between 1979 and 1981, showed that parasite eggs are virtually everywhere, and we must be consuming them without our knowledge. The study showed that over 50% of all the vegetables tested had some parasites. From the samples collected, carrots had the highest percentage at 91.7%. The other parasites and eggs found were 3 *ascaris* eggs, 1,767 larval nematodes (the majority being *rhabditiform*), 175 unidentified eggs, and 44 amoebic cysts!

Even the most careful of washes cannot be 100% guaranteed to remove all parasite presence on *all* food. When we eat out in restaurants, or on holiday, or merely purchase the odd doughnut or sandwich from a fast food outlet, we clearly have no control over the hygiene involved.

Nematodes are just one of the huge number of common parasitic worms that can infest man, animal, insect or plant. They are extremely abundant in nature: a single spadeful of garden soil may contain a million or more nematodes and a bucket of water from a pond usually contains comparable numbers![17] So numerous and widespread are nematodes that N.A. Cobb has written:

If all the matter in the universe except the nematodes were swept away, our world would still be dimly recognizable, and if, as disembodied spirits, we could then investigate it, we should find its mountains, hills, vales, rivers, lakes and oceans represented by a film of nematodes. The location of towns would be decipherable, since for every massing of human beings there would be a corresponding massing of certain nematodes. Trees would still stand in ghostly rows representing our streets and highways. The location of the various plants and animals would still be decipherable and, had we sufficient knowledge, in many cases even their species could be determined by an examination of their erstwhile nematode parasites.[18]

Trichinella spiralis is a human parasite that causes the disease trichinosis, often contracted by eating, amongst other foods, insufficiently cooked pork. Adult

Trichinella worms inhabit the small intestine of numerous species of mammals, among them hogs. To give you a picture of just how small these worms are, and the disproportionately serious damage they can do to humans, it is known that most of the damage of the disease trichinosis occurs during the migration of the larvae, when *half a billion* or more may simultaneously bore through the body after a single infection!

Another human parasite, *Filaria*, is a worm that makes its way to, and lives in, the lymphatic system, where such numbers may accumulate that they block the flow of lymph, causing accumulation of fluid and often enormous swelling of the infected part of the body. Such mechanical blocking of fluid within the body may well be the mechanism behind the food allergy reaction. As I show elsewhere in this book, during such an allergic response, there is reduced bloodflow and we are pretty certain that there is a parasitic presence at the site of the symptom. It seems logical to presume therefore that the parasites enlarge, by gorging on blood, to swell in size, thus creating a physical blockage and reducing the bloodflow.

Even parasitologists' knowledge of parasites is extremely limited. Very little is known about the physiological requirements of the majority of parasites. We don't even know just how many varieties there are – probably millions.

Simply trying to avoid every single parasite and every single egg cannot be the entire answer; they are so prevalent in nature that it would be impossible to do so. Animals cannot avoid them, and under normal everyday circumstances, neither can we. Even if we could, what about all the other people who do not clean their food so scrupulously, yet have *no* illness? They must eat the parasites, and their eggs, yet they are without symptoms. How can this be? That was the next puzzle for me to work on!

Your 'internal environment'

I considered that everyone was approaching the parasite problem from the wrong angle. Whilst I admire Dr. Clark's work enormously and am grateful to it for returning me to the parasite connection I had almost abandoned, I considered that even she must be missing a vital piece of the jigsaw.

Starting the investigation of the problem from a different direction, it seemed inevitable to me that animals in the wild will consume all manner of unwanted bacteria and parasites. This appeared to be normal practice and by Nature's design. But animals in the wild do not have the illnesses that beset modern man. What could be the difference?

What if we were to improve – dramatically – the health of the patient, so that his resistance was strengthened? What if we were to change the patient's 'internal environment' so that it held no attraction for parasites? It is well known that plant parasites do not attack healthy plants. It is also known that parasites tend to settle in those people who are 'under par'.

The only real way, it seemed to me, to enhance the status of someone's health was by correct diet. No drug can permanently restore health – even doctors acknowledge that fact. Drugs may give the appearance of restoring health, temporarily, for instance by alleviating a headache for the duration of the drug's effectiveness. But the drug has not removed the cause, merely temporarily alleviated the symptom.

Take the analogy of a person living on nothing but jelly babies for, say, two years. Assuming the person was still alive at the end of that time, the chances are he would have fatigue, depression, and perhaps bad skin. If he went to the doctor presenting with fatigue, depression, and bad skin, the chances are high that he would walk out of the surgery clutching a prescription for his fatigue, another for his depression, and a third for his skin disorder. Yet the *cause* would have been the appallingly deficient diet, something his doctor had not even considered!

In such a case our patient will continue (no one has told him not to!) his diet of jelly babies. Now his compromised system has toxic drugs as well to deal with. Certainly, these drugs could not restore health to his body. No drug could. It has been shown time and time again that correct diet is the only means of restoring health to the body. Diets like the Gerson therapy are testament to just that fact.

While doctors seem impervious to the link between diet and health, vets are well aware of it. It appears that if you eat natural foods, such as animals in the wild do, even without scrupulous attention to the removal of every possible scrap of parasitic presence, then health will follow.

It is almost certainly our unnatural diets of highly cooked and processed foods – a million miles removed from the diet Nature intended man to eat – that weakens our immune systems and therefore lessens our ability to fend off illness caused by parasites.

One could cite many recoveries brought about by applying purely natural diets, mainly of raw fruits and some cooked vegetables. It all fits: the truly natural diet will restore health to the individual, whose resistance (immunity) will strengthen remarkably, and the disease will retreat into the background as a result.

The parasites reside in the human, obviously attracted to the host's 'internal environment'. By changing his nutrition, it could be that we could alter this environment so that this particular human's body is no longer an attractive habitat for these organisms. If we could achieve this change in the patient's 'internal environment', we would defeat the parasite without directly killing a single one!

If we wanted to eliminate cockroaches from our kitchen, we could tackle the problem in one of two ways.

We could kill each cockroach one by one as they entered the kitchen. Or, we could eliminate every single solitary speck of food in that kitchen. We could remove all the cupboards and kitchen equipment, tile the floor, walls, and ceiling entirely, so that there would no longer be any sustenance for them. For good measure we could further make the kitchen environment extremely cold to further put them off. We could still leave a little gap for them to come in if they wished, but you can rest assured they wouldn't. There would be nothing at all to attract them.

You would have then solved the cockroach problem without killing a single cockroach. You would have altered the environment which attracted them in the first place to one that now holds no attraction whatsoever. You would effectively have found a biological approach to the cockroach problem.

This is what we shall look at next.

8.

The Discovery

If parasites are the problem in the food allergic, what could be wrong with a person's 'internal environment' that the parasites choose that particular body in which to create havoc? There has to be something about the internal environment of the food allergy victim that results in parasites settling in him in the first place.

Unknown to most visitors to my house, which was probably just as well, I had sitting in my fridge, unashamedly beside the food, a pack of 50 million insect parasitic nematodes, *Steinernema feltiae*, which I had obtained in order to study their behaviour. I noted that they would come to life whenever the microscope's substage illuminator was switched on. But I was floundering to capture any other significant aspect of their behaviour. The fact that they responded to light helped me not a jot.

One day, whilst reading a book on biological science, I came across the observation that when amoebas are studied on a slide, if one end is cooled and the other end of the slide is warmed, these parasites will migrate to the warm end.

Amoebas are parasites capable of producing a great deal of illness in man, and, as stated in the last chapter, their presence has been noted in the systems of people with massive food and chemical allergies.

Amoebic dysentery is an illness caused by the organism *Entamoeba histolytica* and spread by contaminated food, water, or flies. If *Entamoeba histolytica* enters into the portal circulation, Amoebic abscess can result. It is not only the liver which can fall prey to such invasion; Amoebic abscesses can affect the lung, brain or spleen.

I read on for a while, then stopped. What was that? What had at first seemed like a relatively mundane and insignificant observation suddenly hit me like a sledgehammer. All at once, after over thirty years of searching, the entire allergy picture fell into place within a matter of seconds! The response of the parasitic amoebas on the microscope slide to temperature change was an absolutely vital clue to their behaviour:

PARASITES ARE TEMPERATURE SENSITIVE!

If my personal food allergy condition was linked to parasites, and if parasites are influenced by temperature, then that explained why my symptoms disappeared when I had a fever! After thirty years of searching, here, finally, was the answer: the temperature of the fever would have been too high for the parasites, thereby inactivating them, at least for the duration of the fever. At that moment I was almost in a state of shock. All at once, other aspects of the food allergy condition just slotted into place.

The fact that the amoebas preferred higher temperatures might not at first sight seem to support my feeling well with a fever. But you have to remember that there is warm and there is hot. Had the temperature kept increasing, the heat would have been too much for them, and would have repelled them.

Was that what the parasites that I kept for study were doing, when I thought they were responding to the light? Were they in fact responding to the *heat* generated by the light under the microscope?

I then remembered that it is standard practice to kill bacteria on food by boiling in water. It is not the banging of their heads against the pan that kills them, nor do they drown. The high temperature destroys them. The other accepted method is to freeze them. Again, we are employing temperature as a means of destruction.

Temperature had to be the answer. I already knew I had a chronically low body temperature. I also knew that even a slight, but chronically-sustained, one degree drop in body temperature can produce all manner of symptoms, both mental and physical. Finally, I also knew that my body temperature consistently climbed during the 7 months I was on the diet until I abandoned it. Therein surely lay the clue to my recovery!

Everything was slotting into place. Had I lasted the course on the Gerson diet, for the 18 months to 2, perhaps 3 years, then the inexorable climb in temperature that I had brought to a halt by abandoning the diet would unquestionably have continued. This explains exactly why people get well on such Nature Cure diets: the normalising of their entire physiological processes, not least their core body temperature, creates an internal environment entirely hostile to parasites.

Furthermore, whilst I was reacting to all foods on the Gerson, near the end of my seven months, I began to notice days when my symptoms, during reactions, were *reducing* in intensity. However, as these good days would soon be followed by bad days, and as I had no real indicator that definite progress was being made (I hadn't analysed the temperature chart at that time), I would soon abandon the diet.

Now, however, the picture was clear; I would simply grit my teeth, suffer the inevitable reactions and continue eating a natural diet. My core body temperature would increase, albeit erratically, and, if the diet was sustained long enough, it would increase to normal, and recovery would result.

The erratic nature of recovery by natural diet is well known and is often the cause of patients giving up prematurely. Encouraged by feeling well one day, the patient despairs at feeling miserable again the next. A return to a junk food diet seems an easy source of solace.

You need only look at the 7-month temperature chart to see just how erratic is the path of recovery. Whilst the progress is not evident from simply glancing at the graph, when it is broken down into temperature climbs per month, then all becomes magnificently clear.

I was thrilled. Before, I would question the wisdom of eating foods that I was reacting to on the diet, and would inevitably abandon the diet through doubt. But with this temperature finding, I could finally see the wisdom of continuing with the natural foods. I could measure my progress by simple daily temperature-taking.

Another of the complaints many patients make when persevering with such long term dietary changes is their recognition that 'nothing seems to be happening' despite their sticking rigidly to instructions.

Now people could record their daily progress and see for themselves the physical evidence that their natural diet was bringing about definite health improvement through the normalisation of their core body temperature.

The improvement almost certainly resulted from the natural cleansing and removal of old encumbrances such a diet would have achieved. The altered internal environment that resulted would be sufficient to render the habitat unsuitable for parasites.

I see them for myself!

I learned more and more about parasites and how to search for them microscopically in my own sputum, blood, urine and faeces, and it wasn't long before I was seeing them with own eyes. When I saw for myself the many parasite eggs coming out of me, I was delighted. For I was trying to connect the food allergy condition to parasites, and although I had been told in America I did have parasites, actually seeing them coming out of your own body is something quite different!

On the back of the cover of this book you can see photographs of parasite eggs eliminated by the author, photographed at 100 x magnification.

CHAPTER EIGHT

Subnormal temperature

Subnormal body temperatures have long been linked to a host of illnesses. More recently Dr. E. Denis Wilson has highlighted this fact in his book *Wilson's Syndrome.*[19]

Dr. Wilson is alert to the fact that people who develop low body temperature most often do so *at a time of trauma in their lives*, which ties in with what we know about the food allergy condition. Many food allergics also recall that it was a death in the family or some other stressful event that triggered off their illness. This is a further clue to the linking of food allergies with mere body temperature.

Dr. Wilson lists the commonest complaints of low body temperature as: fatigue, headaches and migraines, irritability, fluid retention, anxiety and panic attacks, depression, low motivation and ambition, easy weight gain, insomnia, asthma, allergies, heat and/or cold intolerance, and many others.

It should be quickly spotted by the reader that most of these conditions are also in the list of complaints linked to food allergies, which is making the connection between body temperature and food allergies even more certain.

That brain function can be detrimentally affected by a chronically reduced body temperature has also been confirmed. Emanuel Donchin, a psychologist, and Noel K. Marshall, an electrophysicist, both from the University of Chicago, discovered that very slight daily changes in body temperature – one or two degrees below normal – were enough to reduce certain brain responses in test subjects.[20]

Dr. Stephen Langer, in his book *Solved: The Riddle of Illness*, states that a patient even a single degree below the desired 98.6 degrees F. can display all manner of health problems, such as dry, coarse skin, lethargy, depression, mental symptoms, hair loss, weight problems, nervousness, irritability, headaches, palpitations, painful menstruation, difficult breathing, poor memory, and a host of others.

I have had people ask me how a mere *one degree* can be sufficient to incapacitate parasites. Fever is brought about by the body as a very *means* of defeating these organisms. And fever is only just over *one degree* higher than normal body temperature. A degree is a thousand milli-degrees; a parasite may be sensitive to each minute gradation of temperature. I had always considered that if anything was to be the salvation of the food allergic, it could only be diet, even if that diet, in the short term, produced allergic reactions. Sustaining it however, when every mouthful produces a reaction, would require a Herculean amount of faith. For me the necessary willpower came from the evidence of the temperature chart.

Confirmation from the world of gardening

Looking into the temperature connection further, I came across a gardening approach which gave me confirmation that I was on the right track. Gardeners were approaching the problem of plant parasites by a biological route.

The vine weevil is a pest that attacks strawberries. The biological control of the vine weevil is to let loose a nematode worm, a parasite that will attack the vine weevil but not the fruit. However, gardeners observed that the parasite that attacks the vine weevil will not work in soil temperatures below 12 degrees C. By manipulating the control of the soil temperature (the 'environment') they can dictate whether or not parasite activity can take place!

Confirmation from the world of science

I finally found *medical* confirmation of my theory. Micro-organisms can indeed be directly killed by fever in the host animal! To quote from *Pyretics and Antipyretics*:

> ...it was known that syphilis (caused by the parasite *Treponema pallidum*) and gonorrhea (caused by the parasite *Neisseria gonorrhoea*) are heat sensitive and are killed directly by increased temperatures. The basis of treatment before the advent of antibiotics consisted of inducing fevers in these patients using artificial fever caused by injections of BP. The high fevers would subsequently arrest the infecting bacteria.[21]

Thus exists confirmation that parasites can be killed by mere body temperature!

It is known that *Neisseria gonorrhoea* can only survive in a tight range of temperature, that is between 30-39 degrees.C.[22] It is also known that they can be killed at a temperature above that. What goes for one parasite pathogen is almost certain to apply to others; they all have a temperature range in which they best thrive and should that temperature drop, or rise, sufficiently beyond the ideal, that parasite will cease to function.

It is clear to me that the body's response to parasitic infection is to raise the body's temperature to fever level, thus allowing Nature to use her innate wisdom to overwhelm such infestation.

9.

Why the Parasite Connection has been Overlooked

As I looked further into the relationship of parasites to so-called food allergies, and began pooling together information on various related subjects, it became clear why the connection had thus far not been made.

Since orthodox medicine can miss something as highly visible and obvious as a chunk of bread and cheese as being the agent responsible for someone's symptoms, it is hardly surprising that it should miss something invisible to the naked eye as the cause of many health disorders. This is all the more likely when the something invisible is hidden inside the body and is undetectable by X-ray or MRI equipment.

Doctors are dismissive of the food allergy link to illness simply because they haven't been taught it. They will now have to face the fact that another little-studied discipline – parasitology – is also in the picture. And not only has this imprecisely-studied discipline entered the frame, it brings with it a further complicating twist – dietary variations.

Firstly, doctors are frequently unaware of the real physiological mayhem ordinary foods can cause, and secondly, they confuse 'harmless' parasites with 'harmful' ones. What is a 'harmless' parasite in one person can definitely be a 'harmful' one in another! Similarly, what might be a harmless food in one person can definitely be a harmful food in another. Connect it all together and we have the present picture, which links foods and parasites to symptoms of ill health.

Nutritional Medicine has pioneered the recognition of many causes of health disorder which have long baffled orthodoxy. It has shouted loud and hard for over 30 years that foods are intimately linked to everyday disorders. Still orthodox medicine cannot see it, despite countless thousands of people all over the world confirming it for themselves!

Whilst orthodox practitioners still search for chemical concoctions that might ease a headache, we can find the food that causes the headache, eliminate it and thereby end the suffering without drugs.

It is time to move one step further. We can now point to low body temperature due to prolonged poor diet as being instrumental in altering the internal environment of a patient, so that he or she succumbs to unwanted micro-organisms. We can also say that these parasites are responding physically to incoming dietary and chemical influences which result in blood flow interference. This hypoperfusion can, dependent on where in the body it occurs, bring on an entire range of common, everyday disorders.

Not considered

Why are parasitologists not aware of the link to common disorders? Probably for the same reason doctors didn't consider there could be a connection between food and common symptoms: they simply missed it!

Parasitologists have been staring at third-world parasites and linking them with Loa Loa and other exotic illnesses, but they do not appear to have considered that other micro-organisms might be responsible for insomnia, or depression, or fatigue, or arthritis, or any other of the huge number of health disorders that exist in our modern society.

Dieticians didn't know about food allergy – they weren't taught it; nor were doctors or parasitologists. It has been left to Nutritional Medicine to do the research, with little help and considerable resistance from orthodox medicine. We are still uncovering new gems of wisdom relating to widespread health disorders.

I find it almost offensive that orthodoxly trained doctors should consider the field of 'health' to be their domain almost by divine right, when virtually all they can do is dish out toxic drugs and rarely find, far less remove, the true cause. Let us examine the main reasons behind the under-diagnosing of the food–allergy/parasite problem.

The main parasites

There are three main categories of parasites: protozoa (single-celled organisms), platyhelminthes (tapeworms and flukes) and nematodes (hookworms, roundworms, pinworms).[23]

These groups of organisms are exceedingly complex, having multiple groupings and types of organisms within each group.

Protozoa, being single-celled organisms, are relatively crude in morphology compared to other more advanced parasites. They are however able to create problems similar in severity and duration to those of any other parasite group. Indeed, they can affect the body at a cellular level, causing problems in the endocrine, circulatory and gastrointestinal systems.

Platyhelminthes comprise three classes: the trematodes, the cestodes and the turbellaria. All of the trematodes and cestodes are true parasites but only a few of the turbellaria are. The trematodes are normally referred to as flukes, that is flat, leaf-shaped worms.

Some flukes are endoparasitic - that is they live on the outside of their host, most often cold-blooded aquatic vertebrates, while other groups are more complex and occur in all vertebrate groups.[24] They live mainly in the intestines, vascular system and urogenital tract of vertebrates. Note that this ability to remain and thrive in the vascular system of vertebrates is almost certainly highly implicated in food allergy. This is discussed elsewhere in this book in relation to the partial blockage of blood vessels during 'food allergic' reactions.

The cestodes live in the body cavity and intestinal tract of vertebrates, and the trematodes, which lack a digestive system, rely on consuming the partially digested foods from the host itself.

Nematodes is a group that includes many of the well-known worms, such as roundworm, pinworm, hookworm and tapeworm. They are found almost everywhere, not only in man but in all other environments: marine, freshwater, terrestrial and also in plants and animals.[25]

Harmful or harmless?

Parasites are classified as either commensal, symbiotic or pathogenic.

A commensal parasite is thought to live off the host's own diet, give nothing in return, but do no harm.

A symbiotic parasite – a symbiont – is thought to live in 'partnership' with the host, receiving nourishment but rendering service in return. Examples of symbionts are the nitrogen-fixing bacteria of the root nodules of leguminous plants, the cellulolytic bacteria that digest plant food in the intestine of herbivores, and the vitamin-synthesizing bacteria of the human intestine. A pathogen harms its host.

However, according to *Microbial and Parasitic Infection,* these classifications are not as clear cut as once thought. There appears to be considerable confusion as to what are harmful pathogens and what are the harmless commensal parasites. Sometimes there appears to be a change of opinion on this. The classification of organisms as pathogens continues to fluctuate. *The Color Atlas and Textbook of Diagnostic Parasitology* states: 'Few people realize that only a few decades ago *Giardia lambia*, the leading cause of intestinal parasitic infections in the United States, was not considered a pathogen'.[26]

More recently, *Cryptosporidium*, a well-known pathogen in animals, was identified as a human pathogen. Today, a controversy continues about the status of *Blastocystis hominis*. After yeast, *B.hominis* is the most frequently observed organism in faecal samples.[27]

Part of the problem is deciding what are harmful 'pathogens' and what are non-harmful 'commensal' organisms. Many people can harbour pathogens such as *Giardia lambia* or *Entamoeba histolytica* and not have discernible symptoms; conversely, they may produce symptoms from what were considered harmless commensal parasites – *Entamoeba coli* or *Endolimax nana* have been reported.[28]

It is my view that 'commensal' parasites might well be mis-classified and I believe that this is shown in the increasing number of food allergic individuals.

As we are now linking food allergic symptoms to parasites, and we know that there is a blood flow interference during an allergic reaction, which may last an hour or two on average, then we also know that these parasites must be active or in some way change their form or activity for the duration of the 'allergic' reaction.

If the classification of so-called commensal parasites was arrived at using test subjects who were unwittingly food allergic, then there could be a false interpretation of the result, given that parasites can respond to incoming food/chemical substances and appear 'inert' before such exposure.

A parasite might be declared 'commensal,' or harmless, because the test subject might have normal body temperature. The same micro-organism in someone with a *low* body temperature (a food allergic for example) might well prove troublesome and thus be declared 'pathogenic.' It is not the micro-organism so much as the actual patient that should be studied!

If scientists continue to study organisms without taking on board the status of the individual, they will fail to understand the true nature of illness. And if they continue to ignore the food allergy condition - and indeed the effect diet has on the body - they will forever be heading down a blind alley.

A classic example of how food allergies have been misleading doctors for decades is in the taking of blood pressure. It is well known that one food allergic response is the raising or lowering of blood pressure.

Someone with 'normal' blood pressure most of the time can, after a meal, have a raised or lowered reading (recall the author's massive drop in blood pressure during food testing in Rome). If that patient were to eat say, an allergenic breakfast and then go to the doctor's morning surgery, there is every chance that the reading the doctor got would be a distorted one – a temporary false reading.

Similarly, the heart rate can change from a 'normal' beat of 72 per minute to one that races, within minutes of eating a so-called 'ordinary' food, if that person is food allergic. It can also do the reverse, slowing down considerably during a food allergic reaction.

Blood flow too, can change as a result of eating food to which one is allergic. I show elsewhere that there is a blood flow interference during a food allergy reaction that orthodox medicine would have sworn blind could never happen…

All manner of physiological processes will undoubtedly occur in the hour or two period of the duration of a food/chemical allergic reaction. Doctors do not take these temporary, but real, changes into account because they don't know about them.

The food allergy picture described above is a simple but good example of how doctors can unwittingly be misled. The doctor may well be misled in another way during the taking of a patient's blood pressure. If he or she, unfamiliar in food allergies, was taking a patient's blood pressure before the patient consumed cheese, for example, then the reading might be normal. However, after eating the cheese, the blood pressure might well shoot up and the doctor would have a false picture of that patient's blood pressure. The increase is only transient, yet his records will show the patient as hypertensive.

Many such readings might be taken before the doctor is convinced the patient *is* hypertensive, but all it would take for the diagnosis to be confirmed is for the patient to partake of his allergenic meal prior to each visit to the surgery.

A typical, untrained-in-food-allergies doctor would therefore have effectively two misguided pieces of information: Firstly, he would consider the patient as having high blood pressure when in fact, the temporary rise was only an allergic response. Secondly, he would view cheese as harmless when in fact it was harmful to his patient.

The clinical ecologist, however, steeped in the food/chemical allergy phenomenon, would be aware of two things; that the cheese was at that moment in time, 'harmful', and that the blood pressure reading was being influenced only temporarily because of the cheese.

An orthodox doctor instructed in the food allergy condition might be brave enough to admit his error and re-classify the cheese as harmful (at least in that patient).

Of course we now have the other problem. An organism carried by one person might well do him no harm, but the same organism carried by another person may well create physiological havoc. This is the situation we observe with HIV positive patients – one does not develop full-blown AIDS, whilst another does. The same organism is at work, but the two people are obviously different. It is fairly probable that it is the body temperature, the patient's 'internal environment', which makes all the difference.

Could one HIV-positive patient be viewed as carrying a 'commensal' parasite because it creates 'no harm' in him, whilst his friend, who is also HIV-positive but with the full-blown illness, be considered to be carrying a 'pathogenic' HIV?

Confusion in classification and lack of knowledge of the true extent of the nature of parasites must go some way to explaining why doctors are simply unaware of the connection between them and so-called ordinary health disorders.

10.

Fever: Friend or Foe?

Doctors have long been in doubt as to whether fever is a friend or an enemy. One thing they all do agree on is that fever is a sign of illness. The mechanics of fever are little understood but it is recognised that many physiological processes speed up considerably at this time.

It is known that invading micro-organisms can invoke fever. Whilst doctors recognise that fever occurs during infection, they are unclear as to whether or not the fever has brought about the infection or the infection has resulted in a fever. It appears clear to me now that fever is the body's own mechanism by which to combat such invasion.

There are books entirely devoted to 'Pyrexia' – fever – and the only thing that is clear after reading them is that science still has not made its mind up as to whether fever is a good or bad process.

The normal body temperature of 37 degrees C. (98.6 degrees F.) exists in health, but this figure is not very far away from the maximum temperature (42 degrees C.) that can be endured for hours or days without bringing about permanent damage.

Dangers also exist in lowered temperatures. From the hypothermic levels of temperature that can bring about frostbite and death, all the way up to the higher range of temperature that is hyperthermia, which can also result in death, various degrees of health can exist.

37 degrees C. is ideal. Any change from that, whether up or down, can have a bearing on your health. And while a relatively short drop in temperature – as may exist in the morning before you rise – may be harmless, a chronic and sustained drop in temperature can bring about all manner of undesirable symptoms.

Whilst humans have a built-in fever-producing system for times of illness, Kluger found that sick lizards automatically sought out hot environments in order to raise their body temperatures to fever level when they became ill.[29]

It appears that fever is part of the body's defence mechanism and it seems that whilst science, even today, argues whether fever is friend or foe, Nature, in all her wisdom, has known since time began how to produce a natural defence against invading organisms. The fever response is provoked as a direct result of such invasion.

My own personal experiences of fever have always been positive, inasmuch as my specific symptoms of food allergy have deserted me during such a time. I have always welcomed fevers for that very reason.

When radical changes in diet are undertaken, such as with a Nature Cure approach, there often occurs, several weeks into such a diet, a 'healing crisis'. That is a time when the temperature often rises. There may be nausea, and even depression and fatigue may appear. But, unlike orthodox doctors, who are often dismayed at the presence of a fever and feel they 'have to do something' to reduce it, naturopathic doctors and nutritional medicine practitioners welcome such a crisis and recognise it as a vital first step to recovery. Once the fever abates, more often than not the patient experiences an improvement in wellbeing.

Temperature in disease

The role of temperature in disease is a fascinating one. The crayfish has been shown to seek out warmer temperatures when infected with bacteria. Fish, amphibians and reptiles also respond to the invasion of live bacteria by seeking out warmer ambient temperatures and raising their body temperatures to fever levels in order to combat such infections. Birds and most mammals also respond with a fever to live bacteria. *Pyretics and Antipyretics* states:

> The question of the beneficial value of fever to an infected animal has been the subject of speculation and investigation for many years. Fevers could be beneficial to an animal in two ways:
>
> (1) The high body temperatures of fever could exceed the temperature beyond which the infectious micro-organism could live and thereby directly kill it.
>
> (2) Indirectly by affecting one or several biochemical, cellular or humoral components of the body which in turn destroy the micro-organism. This effect could, in turn, involve a change that directly destroyed the micro-organism or a change that depleted an essential substrate of it.[28]

Whilst science still knows comparatively little about the behaviour of parasites, it recognises that the host's internal environment has to be suitable in order for that organism to live, reproduce, and thrive. Current knowledge of the preferred temperature range of parasites is extremely limited and much guesswork is involved.

To quote from *Microbial and Parasitic Infections* (Edward Arnold, London 1993: p38):

A pathogen must be able to multiply in or on the host's tissues. This means that the host's tissues must supply appropriate nutrients, atmospheric conditions and temperature for the pathogen's growth. Here we can see in broad outline the facts which determine the host ranges of all pathogens and indeed of all parasites, but we can fill in very few of the details.

Tosca's fever

The following tale is related by Dr. Virginia Vetrano, who studied under Dr. Herbert Shelton, the world's foremost practitioner in fasting. She knew the importance of a fever in restoring health and the manner in which she handled it when her child was ill should be a lesson to us all. I thank Dr. Vetrano for her permission to use this lovely story.

Our daughter, Tosca, who was only 18 months old at the time, had suddenly developed a fever for the first time in her life. There were no symptoms of a cold. She never had one. There was only a fever, which began with a flushing of her cheeks, and a listlessness that was uncommon to her. The fever wasn't high, but it was sufficient to cause anxiety and convert her usual bubbling personality to a quiet solemnity. The personality change was so radical that it was a great shock to us.

Having learned of Hygiene (fasting/diet) at the age of 18, and having devoured each *Hygienic Review* as it came to me every month, and having avidly studied Dr. Shelton's books thoroughly, I naturally put the feverish child on a complete fast. I had no fear. I had reared her Hygienically. She had been breast fed for nine months, after which nothing but unpasteurised milk and fresh fruit juices passed her lips as long as I was around.

Occasionally, when I wasn't around, a doting relative feeling Tosca was being deprived, would slip her a piece of chocolate but otherwise her diet and other factors of her life were always in accord with her anatomical and physiological age.

I had all the confidence in the world that in a few days Tosca would be well again. But, my husband, having never studied Hygiene, was worried.

At first, he left matters in my hands because I was so very confident, and seemed to know just what to do.

The evening of the first day of her fast she vomited bile. The second day she slept almost all the time, waking only occasionally. She wouldn't drink much water, but I gave some to her in a bottle every now and then, just to see if she was thirsty. She would take the bottle and begin to drink, but, after tasting the water, she would make a disgusted looking face, and push the nipple out of her mouth with her tongue.

Her fever dropped but it was still a little high, and by the third day my husband and all my in-laws began to show concern. 'I wonder what's wrong with her?' they'd ask, and 'shouldn't we do something?'.

Tosca's great aunt, who loved her dearly, came to see her every day and would sit for long hours saying 'Elle, n'est pas dans son assiette' over and over again. I wished I could tell her to hush up. We all knew that 'she wasn't like her usual self.' But I understood this as great concern and held my tongue.

Tosca was on the fifth day of her fast – five days mind you of not eating at all – and still feverish. This is when my husband began to doubt Hygienic care. Like most people, he expected miracles. He became increasingly nervous and worried, and began pacing the floor. He went to his aunt's for a while. I don't know what discussion took place, but evidently they had upset him still more, for he looked worse when he returned.

After nervously smoking for a while, he took another walk and then came back in, to pace the floor again. Then he went out again, and returned in 15 minutes with the same frightened and worried look. Finally by late afternoon, when we again took Tosca's temperature and she still had fever, he could no longer control himself. He could hold just so much steam. He yelled, the threat at me, slammed the door, and went out for another walk.

How fortunate I was. I knew what Nature could do. How peaceful it is to know the laws of life. I knew that the living organism could right what was wrong better when left alone than when meddled with, but he had no such faith. Neither did his family, or they wouldn't have been so frightened.

I stayed with Tosca while she slept peacefully, as do all sick children when cared for Hygienically. But, how I wished Nature were not so slow! I was getting impatient myself because of my husband's threat and his family's behaviour. I was just as concerned as they were, and it had been difficult to maintain my cool, while others were wringing hands and pacing floors. But I had to. If I had once shown alarm and a lack of confidence, Tosca would have immediately been rushed to a doctor, and drugged against my will. I could not bear the thought of this, after having heard the evil effects of drugs.

Finally, the evening of the fifth day, her temperature dropped to normal. How excited and thrilled and gloriously thankful I was! She was well and I wouldn't have to fight off my husband's threat the next day. I couldn't wait until he came back from his walk to tell him the good news. He was so relieved when he heard the news that he took Tosca in his arms, and held her closely for a while. He wanted to feed her right away, and wanted to run down for some oranges immediately. Then I disappointed him yet again, because I said 'No.' Tosca had to fast until the next morning. I had read in Dr. Shelton's care of children, to feed too soon after fever drops is to bring it back again. So he agreed to wait until morning, but he got the oranges that night so I'd have them early the next day.

The stony silence, the edgy nerves, the impatience, and the worried looks of my in-laws when Tosca had fever, outwardly portrays the prevailing fear of fever. The very means the body has of coping with excess waste, bacteria or their toxins, and other poisons, frightens people because of a lack of understanding of it. Their fear is misplaced. They should fear the causes of fever, not the fever itself, which is the body's means of defence, cleansing, and repair. It is a remedial process and not an offensive one.

Fear of fever is still with us, and almost every time I lecture, I am asked 'How do you bring a fever down?' and 'Don't very high fevers damage the brain?' and other similar questions intimating that fever is dangerous. I always answer that fever will come down of its own accord when the body has eliminated the cause of the fever. No matter what occasions the fever, the fever is always beneficial, and never harmful.

Although the medical profession in general still maintains their fear of fever, some doctors do understand that it can be beneficial and sometimes try to bring on an artificial fever with drugs. In Nature, fever appears when all parts of the body are ready to handle this important condition. Artificial fevers, however, do not comply with Nature and very rarely achieve the desired results.

It is a common belief that one should 'feed a fever'. But Nature knows best. More often than not appetite entirely disappears. Instead of force-feeding the patient in the mistaken belief that this will endow him with strength, one should listen to Nature and recognise that she has removed appetite for a reason: all energies are required to battle with the invading organisms and should not be diverted unnecessarily into pushing piles of food through 30 feet of tubing.

My last book *Allergies Make You Fat* – now re-published under the title *Discover Your Hidden Food Allergies* – showed that during a fasting experiment on myself, my body temperature increased during a fast each and every morning, until I ate. Then the reading on the next morning showed a drop in temperature. Several variations of that experiment produced the same result, clearly indicating that eating in some way interferes with the production of body heat.

A noted British doctor, A. Rabagliati, M.A., M.D., F.R.C.S. Edin., applied fasting to many of his patients, with remarkable success. He observed that patients who might have had a sub-normal core body temperature for many years, saw their temperature climb during the fast, inevitably reaching normal by the conclusion of a long fast. At that time, more often than not, the patient would recover from his symptoms.

Rabagliati's experience with fasting and body temperature is commonly observed amongst practitioners who are experienced at employing such 'negative-nutrition' techniques.

This further points to the deprival of appetite during fever as being crucial to recovery. If, as we have shown, stopping eating (fasting) can result in a climb in core body temperature, and eating can bring about a drop, then the physician or anxious relative who encourages the patient to eat when he has no appetite, during a fever, will be obstructing the rise in temperature crucial to bringing about the very defeat of invading micro-organisms.

It is clear, therefore, that if the body does not demand food during a fever, no food whatsoever should be given! By all means drink as much water as is desired, but if a true appetite does not exist, it is wrong to insist on eating. The body will recover and be all the stronger for it, if one doesn't eat during a fever.

Examples of heat as a means of destroying parasites have long existed

It appears we have unwittingly been using temperature control for some considerable time when it comes to micro-organisms. Outbreaks of the bacteria *Giardia* occur frequently in the United States. Between 1979 and 1990 over 15,000 cases were reported in Pennsylvania alone. What instructions were given to avoid infection, and kill such parasites? Boil all water! *Giardia* is a water-borne organism so small that 8,000 can fit onto the head of a pin. The instructions were to boil water before drinking it and thereby kill the organism.

What does boiling the water do? As I state elsewhere, the micro-organisms do not drown in the water. They do not die from their heads being knocked on the side of the pan. It is simply the change of temperature that kills them.

Boiling has long been recognised as a way of defeating bacteria and that ties in perfectly with the subject of this book. Another method of destroying such organisms has also been long known: freezing. Again, it is the change of temperature that is responsible for the end of such parasites, not the darkness of the freezer.

Pinworms are parasites which are notorious for infecting children. Dr. Leo Litter, a paediatrician from Connecticut, recommends 'superheating' the home to 95 degrees F. for a day. Dr. Litter states that this is the most effective way to kill embryos in the eggs. Notice that he does not say to heat the home for a mere hour, but for a whole day. That tells us that a sustained change in temperature is required to end the parasites' existence and that a single blast might not be enough. Again, however, we have the recognition that you can destroy parasites by mere temperature change.

11.

You Can Defeat Hereditary Illness

We know that 'allergies' are inherited. We recognise that there are 'inherited tendencies' for an allergic disease such as asthma to run in the family. But the real truth seems to be that, as parasites are involved in allergic activity, it is the parasitic organisms that can be passed to the offspring from the parents.

Doctors always appear misty-eyed when talking about some illness or other that is hereditary. There is an aura of mysticism about diseases that are 'passed down', with no good explanation other than 'if your grandfather had it, that'll explain it'. Such a hazy explanation is the best attempt doctors can give for the phenomenon that is hereditary illness.

Fear pervades families when there is a serious illness or deformity 'somewhere in the line'. The passing down is well recognised within families. But are we giving the phenomenon more respect than it deserves? Might there not be a relatively simple explanation?

I suggest there is something you can do about it, something very, very effective, to prevent yourself or your children 'inheriting' a condition that exists within your family. Even if you, or your children, are 'confirmed carriers'.

Treponema pallidum is a parasite responsible for syphilis. Children can be born with congenital syphilis. *Treponema pallidum* is a spiral-shaped bacterium – a spirochaete – that is a well known 'hereditary' parasite.

But remember that it is a physical organism, a parasite that has entered one human and passed down through to the next generation. There is nothing 'mystical' in that. It is a physical passing between body fluids, a mere journey of the micro-organism within a fluid medium, swimming from one place (mother's body) to another place (foetus's body).

This simple explanation of how one disease passes down through the ranks of a family can also provide us with the clue to *most* hereditary disease.

If, as I contend, far more diseases than previously considered are a direct result of parasitic infestation, then could this not be an explanation of the miasmic taints that appear to exist with other 'hereditary' diseases, such as asthma, or mental illness?

Orthodox medicine has overlooked food allergy as the cause of much illness, and it has overlooked the organisms that appear to work hand-in-hand with that 'cause' of illness So, is it not almost mandatory that they will have missed this highly likely explanation for the 'hereditary' way in which the organism is transported from host to the next generation?

If syphilis can be passed down from one generation to the next, why not all parasitic diseases? Do not allow the fact that syphilis is sexually transmitted divert you from the true picture. In congenital syphilis we witness a micro-organism invading a man; he passes it to another human, who passes it to another. No magic. No mysticism. Simple swimming! As our bodies are about 70% water, what better method of transport can any parasite have?

Food allergics are in such a state because of parasites. Accept this and you have the 'hereditary' package neatly tied up. To prevent it running through your family, you have to drive the parasitic infestation from your own system and that of any children you have, by dietary reform. Just as Pottenger's cats' offspring turned their health around by improved nutrition.

It was only in the early 20th century that widespread food processing and food adulteration began. With it, the incidence of all manner of illness has shot up. Our grandparents', our parents', and our own diets have been playing a massive part in shaping the state of health of all of us today. Our diets play a part in the health of our offspring as well, as we have seen with the offspring's health in the Pottenger cats' experiment. By eating correctly – that is, natural-ly – we have the chance to turn our own health around. If we don't, each future generation will suffer more and more illness.

Many other diseases are medically accepted as being of parasitic origin and also known to be able to be passed down through this watery route. Meningitis is one. HIV is another. Someone can carry the *Neisseria meningitis* parasite without displaying any symptoms at all. Another person can carry it and devel-op illness. To quote from *Microbial and Parasitic Infection* (p218):

Most people who acquire *N. meningitis* in this way carry it in their upper respiratory tracts for a period but suffer no ill effects. However, a small pro-portion of those who become colonized subsequently develop invasive infection. The reason why only some people are susceptible to infection is not known, but responsibility appears to lie with the immune system, and there may be a relationship with HLA type.

I believe that the reason some people are not affected adversely by the parasite is simply because their core body temperature is high enough – they are healthy enough – to take care of such unwanted bacterial invasion.

The Pottenger Cats' experiment and other diet research has shown quite clearly that not only is the health of the animal dependent upon their diet, but that their offspring's health is critically linked to their parent's dietary habits. It should go without saying that this dietary implication will also translate to humans. Our parent's diets will undoubtedly have been important in our development. Since the diet of the parents plays a critical part in the health of the offspring, it is clear that each of us will be born with a different 'status' of health.

That status will play a part in the future health of our child, and the child's own diet will complement what he was given at birth. The picture of the food allergic therefore will be something like this:

Status at Birth

(Likely) Highly processed diet
causing
Subnormal core body temperature
causing
Ideal parasitic 'Internal environment'
causing
Parasitic infestation, often after stress

Patient eats allergenic meal
causing
Parasitic activity
causing
Blood vessel (or lumen) closing due to 'simple' blockage
causing
Hypoperfusion at site of parasites

SYMPTOMS

To Reverse Illness:

Patient adopts unprocessed, *natural* diet
leading to
Gradual increase to normal core body temperature
leading to
'Internal environment' becoming hostile to Parasites
leading to
Parasitic activity (Allergic reaction) ceasing
leading to

End of Symptoms

It is well known that micro-organisms can lie dormant for many years and then 'spring' into action for no apparent reason bringing about symptoms of ill health. To quote again from *Microbial and Parasitic Infection* (p61):

Failure of the host's defences to eliminate a pathogen soon after its arrival may result in persistent active disease. Often however, there is a balance between the pathogen and the defences, and the infection may remain asymptomatic (latent) for many years but turn into active disease again when the balance is shifted in favour of the pathogen.

The same book states (p63):

An increase in body temperature is a very common host response to infection. It may *well be* protective in some circumstances, e.g., by providing an environment too warm for optimal growth of the pathogen (micro-organism).

We know that the incidence of 'allergies' and all manner of illnesses has increased dramatically in recent decades. As our nutrition has never in the history of mankind been so badly altered and interfered-with, it should be no surprise nor coincidence that our poor long term eating habits have now caught up with us and that our 'civilised' society is now beset with widespread ill health.

Target organs

We know also that micro-organisms such as viruses or parasites show marked tissue– and organ-specificity, e.g., for salivary glands (mumps virus), for the breast or kidneys (cytomegalo virus) or for the respiratory tract (measles). *Microbial and Parasitic Infection* (p43) recognises that:

the mechanisms of disease production by these more complex parasites are themselves extremely complex. . . . The site occupied by the parasite is important; if this is its usual habitat, the resulting disease may be relatively minor compared with the effects produced by the same parasite in unusual sites – e.g. a few *Paragonimus* eggs in the brain may cause far more serious effects than a much larger number in their more usual situation in the lungs. The severity of disease caused depends not only on the number of parasites present, but also on the physiological state of the host(s). It goes

on: 'Any lowering of general health predisposes to more serious consequences of parasite attack'.[31]

Again we see the standard acceptance that a 'lowered' state of health can pre-
dispose to parasitic attack. As a lowered state of health will almost certainly co-
exist with a subnormal temperature, orthodox medicine and this book are
entirely in agreement...

This recognition that parasites will invade only those with a lowered state of
health is well known. To quote a Californian organic gardener: 'Bugs don't
attack healthy plants.' And to quote from *Microbial and Bacterial Infection* (p27);
'A few bacterial species are virtually always pathogenic to man: They are not
found in healthy individuals.'

It could well be the case that 'bugs' do attack healthy individuals but healthy
individuals' core body temperature somehow arrests their activity so that they
no longer pose a damage to their host, as in the case of an HIV-positive person displaying no symptoms, or the carrier of the meningococcal virus being
only the carrier and not developing the full-blown symptoms.

Parasites and the allergy connection

Throughout this book there is sufficient information to show that the food
allergy condition (which is no more than the linking of a diet connection to
your symptoms, whatever they are) and parasites are connected. We also are
aware that 'allergies' are hereditary.

The following is a superb example of how parasites can be in the body yet
show no symptoms until after eating. This is much the same as a food allergy
sufferer who might be host to parasites but not display symptoms until after
eating, when his discomfort will last about an hour generally.

Human Parasitology (p29) states: Toxocara spp.: A case was reported by Rodan
and Buckley (1969) of a child, aged 4, who suffered from frequent epigastric
pains, lasting half to one hour, often connected with meals, for 4 weeks, prior
to vomiting a T. cati worm.[32]

12.

Parasites – The Hidden Epidemic?

The list of health problems linked to parasites is large. However, my feeling is that there exists a gross under-estimation of the true extent to which parasites are culpable.

Many common illnesses have been shown to be of parasitic origin. Could it be that *most* common complaints, from arthritis to depression, from migraine to insomnia, previously thought not to have any connection with invading parasites, can in fact be manifestations of an undiagnosed parasitic presence?

We know invading micro-organisms can interfere with our health. Illness by invasion of organisms is known throughout biology. It is known that plants can become 'ill' – can become diseased – through parasitism. Animals can be parasitised and display symptoms of distress and ill health. Birds can become ill when infested with parasitic organisms. Even insects, so small they can barely be seen, can become victim to even smaller organisms – parasites – and have their health destroyed.

Throughout life on the planet tiny parasitic organisms can cause ill health. A good number of human illnesses are instigated by parasites. We have already recognised some links. We also know that the discipline of parasitology is ill-defined and in its infancy. But we seem to stop short of pointing the finger at such organisms as bearing responsibility for a whole further range of illnesses.

We rarely consider symptoms of depression or mental illness as being caused by an invading organism. But we should. Because it can happen. *Candida albicans* can cause mental symptoms, for one.

Let us consider some known parasites and the illness they can produce in humans and compare this vast array of health problems to the vast array of health problems put down to 'food allergies'. Remember that there are many parasites of humans yet to be discovered and, more importantly, linking them to symptoms is quite another skill!

All of the following symptoms can be caused by parasites. Whilst parasitic activity may not be present every time that these symptoms appear, the possiblity of their presence should *never* be ignored.

Just some of the conditions which can be caused by parasites

Asthma[33]
Rheumatic fever[34]
Arthritis[35,36,37,38]
Hyperactivity/
Attention Deficit Disorder[39]
Alzheimer's[40]
Epilepsy[41,42]
Headaches[43]
Mental confusion[44]
Urticaria[45]
Nervousness[46]
Migraine[47]
Weight loss[48]
Weight gain[49,50]
Vascular Disorders[51]
Thrush[52]
Mouth Ulcers[53]
Food Allergy[54]
Depression[55]
Personality changes[56]
Chronic fatigue[57,58]
Bloating[59]
Conjunctivitis[60]
Oedema[61]

Eczema[62]
Osteomylitis[63]
Cystitis[64]
Irritable Bowel Syndrome
(IBS)[65]
Sore throats[66]
Impetigo[67]
Acne[68]
Skin infections[69]
Warts[70]
Abdominal pain[71]
Burning pain in penis
on urinating[72]
Jaundice[73]
Hepatitis[74]
Anaemia[75]
High Blood Pressure[76]
Heartbeat, irregular
(arrhythmia)[77]
Myalgia[78]
Dermatitis[79]
Urinary tract infections[80]
Anorexia[81]

These are just some of the varieties of ill health that can be brought about by the presence of parasites.

Parasites and common symptoms

Gastric and duodenal ulcers have long been the cause of much distress in humans, yet it was only as recently as 1983 that a connection to a parasite was made. An Australian scientist shouted loud and hard that he had made the discovery that a spiral-shaped micro-aerophillic organism was involved in these stomach disorders. His findings were dismissed by orthodox medicine. But eventually they did accept his findings and the responsibility of *Helicobacter pylorus* for much human misery was finally recognised.

Candida Albicans is another parasite that has become well known only relatively recently. Although properly studied as mycology, micro-organisms such as fungi are still classed as parasites.

Candida is in everyone. But not everyone is harmed by its presence. And because everyone has Candida, it is rarely considered as being responsible for some very common health disorders. It appears that although we all may be host to such fungi, not all of us allow it to run out of control. The long-term use of antibiotics has been linked to the proliferation and overgrowth of this fungus and it is when that happens that trouble arises.

Candida (pronounced kan-did-ah not kan-deed-ah) can be responsible for many common conditions such as migraine, irritability, depression, acne, cystitis, vaginitis, thrush, bloating and constipation, amongst other conditions.[82]

From that list the migraine symptom in particular jumps out at me. There is strong evidence to suggest that migraine is caused by a blood flow disturbance. It is also a favourite food-allergy disorder. Now we recognise it can be produced by a parasite. The four-way link up is again there for all to see: food allergies, parasites, blood flow and symptoms…

Consider the irritability symptom from the above list. If the condition refuses to respond to medication, a patient might well be referred to psychiatrists in order to fathom out what dark childhood secret lies at the back of the mental anguish that manifests as irritability. A mere physical organism – a parasite – can be responsible, rather than some dark childhood secret!

Epilepsy

We know that there is a blood flow interruption in epilepsy. We also know that parasites can cause epilepsy, by their presence in the brain.[83]

It is known that the presence of parasites in the brain can cause many neurological disorders and can cause epilepsy[84]. However, it is very likely that 'run of the mill' epileptic events where the patient at his workplace has a fit and then recovers will almost certainly not be considered of parasite origin.

The incident will simply be classed as a 'fit' or a 'seizure' and the appropriate drugs given. After all, even if an X-ray was taken there and then, parasites would not show on the image.

Chlamydia is another parasite that is coming to the fore. Responsible for infertility, it is estimated to exist in up to 10% of the British population. It is the most commonest sexually-transmitted disease in Britain and it is expected to affect over 100,000 young women in the immediate future.[85]

Chlamydia is capable of creating clinical mayhem. There are three strains of

Chlamydia, serologically identical to each other but micro-biologically different: *Chlamydia pneumoniae*, *Chlamydia psittaci* and *Chlamydia trachomatis*. All are parasites, and they cause symptoms such as pneumonia, bronchitis, eye infections, genital tract infections, trachoma, urethritis (non-gonococcal), and inflammations in many other organs including the liver.

Although considered a sexually-transmitted disease, Chlamydia can be transmitted by airborne means.[86] Giardia is the most commonly reported parasite in Britain. This organism attaches itself to the wall of the small intestine by means of a sucking disc, and a layer of Giardia can cover the intestinal villi. Giardia is transmitted in cyst form (a dormant stage of a parasite) through food and water routes or even from animal faeces containing the Giardia cysts.

Symptoms initially can include diarrhoea, bloating, nausea, foul-smelling gas and abdominal cramps. Chills, belching and headache may also be present. The symptoms may diminish, but Giardia can also attach itself to the bile ducts of the liver, exhibiting symptoms identical to gall bladder disease.

Prolonged infection with Giardia can cause damage to the intestinal villi producing problems such as chronic iron deficiency, anaemia, vitamins A and B-12 deficiencies, folic acid deficiency, fat malabsorption, lactose intolerance and low serum calcium.[87]

Clearly there is the possibility of clinical confusion in this list of symptoms. Anyone presenting with symptoms of B-12 or folic acid deficiency would usually be treated accordingly with supplementation when, at the back of it all, is a parasite responsible for such ill health; the nutrient deficiency is only a secondary symptom and not the primary one.

Other Illnesses

It is becoming very clear that many common diseases which have never before been considered of parasitic origin, have indeed such an organism implicated.

Arthritis, the cause of which has baffled medical science for centuries, is almost certainly linked to parasites.[88,89,90]

Lyme Disease was 'discovered' in Lyme, Connecticut, USA. The symptoms are identical to arthritis. Is this another case of a common disorder now being linked to a parasite? Almost certainly. Arthritis is a condition well known to be triggered by foods, in other words a food allergy condition.

Scientists in Boston, USA, have now found a parasite – a microbe – in the brains of Alzheimer's sufferers and this may be another case of a relatively 'common' but distressing illness being linked to a living organism invading the host, the parasite invasion not being recognised until very recently.[91]

One of the most common parasites detected in stool samples is *Blastocystis hominis* which can cause 'unexplained' symptoms of nausea, stomach pain, diarrhoea and general malaise.

Toxoplasmosis can be passed to humans from cats. Breathing the dust that contains the infected eggs in the cats' faeces is one way of becoming infected. Another means of getting the condition is eating undercooked or improperly cooked meat such as beef, lamb, or pork.

Toxoplasmosis is one of those diseases that can lay 'dormant' in the human and cause no symptoms. When symptoms do appear, they may take the form of fever, headache, chills and fatigue.

Ascaris lumbricoides is the most common parasite in the world and it is estimated that approximately 1 billion people have the worm. Once the adult worm develops in the human system, it can travel around the body, ending up in the heart, lungs or liver. A host of symptoms is linked to Ascaris, including, in children, nervousness, asthma, poor appetite, failure to thrive, coughing and wheezing, and allergic reactions. Here again are common 'allergy' symptoms linked to a parasite: asthma, nervousness and allergic reactions all capable of being caused by *Ascaris lumbricoides*.

Meningitis is another parasite-produced illness that causes fear in mothers in all modern societies. But whilst many of us can be 'carriers' of the parasite, not all of us develop the illness that is associated with it.

The position of the 'carrier' who does not develop the full-blown illness has been addressed elsewhere in this book, but it is worth repeating when we are discussing illnesses such as meningitis. My opinion is that the reason for this will relate to the core body temperature, or 'internal environment' of the victim. If the host's body temperature is high enough to inactivate the microorganism, no symptoms of meningitis will appear. But if his diet and lifestyle become so chronically poor that his core body temperature falls below 98.6 degrees F., then it seems reasonable to deduce that will be when he will develop the full-blown illness.

Similarly with HIV and AIDS. Many people are HIV-positive, that is, they are carriers of the virus but do not develop full-blown AIDS. Again, it is my belief that, if the body temperature of those carriers who have been infected is in the normal range, they will not develop the illness, but if the HIV organism enters the body of someone with a low body temperature, the illness will take hold. However, if the HIV-positive sufferer who has no symptoms sustains a life-style of poor diet/alcohol/smoking long enough, his health (and temperature) will gradually decline and that may then trigger the full-blown illness.

The creeping, flesh-eating parasite that was the scourge of hospitals in the mid 1990s, where surgeons watched helplessly as flesh on their patients almost visibly disappeared, is another horrific instance of a parasite making good when the conditions were ripe. Parasites are known to favour the bodies of weakened animals; there is no human more at risk than one who is lying on an operating table with his insides exposed to the open world. It will be almost certain that the temperature of such a body will be considerably below that of a normal human being.

As our diets become more and more artificial and unnatural, it will be inevitable that our core temperature – and our vitality – will reduce. Sooner or later we will become prey to more and more parasitic infections. That the health of populations in 'civilised' Westernised countries like Britain and the USA grows worse by the year, ties in exactly with what one would expect as a result of our appalling nutrition.

The number of children presenting with asthma in a recent study was twice that of eight years earlier, according to a study at Leicester University which involved researchers questioning parents of 2,600 pre-school children. *Asthma News* reported that while 11% of pre-school children had been diagnosed with asthma in 1990, this figure had risen to almost 20% in 1998.

Yet the clue to asthma has to be in the finding that laboratory workers with the parasite Ascaris developed urticaria and asthma![92]

Long lived parasites

Parasites might be microscopic in size, but their effect on human health can be immense, even to the extent of bringing the host's life to an end.

A tiny parasite on its own might pose no threat, but when you remember that the most common parasite in the world, *Ascaris lumbricoides*, will produce up to 200,000 (two hundred thousand) eggs in a single day, then they really no longer are the insignificant presence that you might think![93]

Not only can they have a disproportionately adverse affect on one's health but they can have a seriously out-of-proportion lifespan in our bodies. Syphillis itself can exist in our bodies for upwards of 30 years and other diseases 50 years or longer. The truth is, science knows extremely little about the lifespans and indeed, physiological requirements, of much of the parasitic world. *From Microbial and Parasitic Infection* (p49/50):

> The usual incubation period from the date of infection to the onset of lymphangitis is 5 to 18 months, but periods of up to *twenty years* have been recorded.

A single Strongyloide can remain in a human for up to 30 years.[94] *Taenia saginata* – beef tapeworms – can live in the human for up to 25 years, with only one worm at a time inhabiting the system.[95] From *Modern Parasitology:*[96]

> The schistosomula effectively disguised as host, and therefore immunologically invisible, can migrate around the body and eventually enter blood vessels associated with the gut or bladder where they mature into adults. Adults live for about 5 years during which time they evade immunological attack but produce thousands of eggs, some of which lodge in tissues including the liver.

With an ongoing production line of many thousands of offspring, each capable of living for 5 years, it is no wonder man, or animal for that matter, can be ill their entire lives! From *Microbial and Parasitic Infection:*[97]

Onchocerca volvulus is a parasite disease, transmitted by blood-sucking insects. They penetrate human skin via the insect bite, and undergo development as they migrate around the body for the next year! To quote once more from *Miocrobial and Parasitic Infections:* [98]

> Some viruses are able to evade or interfere with host defence mechanisms and remain in the body for long periods. Some, such as polyoma and adenoviruses, can remain latent in this way for *many years* without any obvious effect on the host. Others – notably the herpes simplex and varicella–zoster viruses mentioned above in connection with nervous systems infections – can persist in a *latent* non-infectious form but may be reactivated from time to time to produce symptomatic and transmissible infections; such reactivation is usually associated with impairment of general health or immunity.

One wonders if that 'latent non-infectious form' is simply a euphemism for saying that the organism is arrested in its activity by increased body temperature? And that the 'reactivation' is simply what occurs in the host when, through long term poor diet, his body temperature reduces?

The criticality of temperature

It is well established in medicine that a reduced temperature, such as that found in hypothyroidism (underactive thyroid) can result in a host of symptoms.

The normal temperature for humans is considered to be 98.6 degrees.F., with a slightly lower reading in the morning and often a slightly increased reading at night. However, even a drop of a single degree can result in many conditions of ill health. Emanuel Donchin, a psychologist, and Noel K. Marshall, an electrophysicist, from the University of Illinois, discovered that even a small change of 1 or 2 degrees below normal can reduce certain brain responses in test subjects.[99] They discovered that such a reduced body temperature can be responsible for slowing down our movements or thought processes.

In hypothermia – a severe reduction in body temperature – brain wave peaks are markedly delayed, yet when the temperature of such patients is raised to normal, the brain waves speed up and become normal. It stands to reason that a lesser reduction in temperature would have a lesser, but nevertheless identifiable, impact, on brain function.

Donchin and Marshall have recommended that before doctors arrive at the conclusion that a patient has irreversible brain damage, they should consider the body temperature!

At the University of Leiden in the Netherlands, one scientist, G. A. Kerkhof discovered that test subjects produced their best performances when presented with tasks when their body temperature peaked, and that their worst performances occurred when their body temperature was lowered.[100] These results tend to explain why some people categorise themselves as 'morning' or 'evening' people, as body temperature can alter during the day.

Chronically reduced body temperatures are far more prevalent than normally considered. Dr. Broda Barnes, a much respected researcher into hypothyroidism, after whom the Barnes Basal Temperature Test is named, estimates that no less than 40 percent of the adult population of the United States suffers from an often unrecognised subnormal body temperature.[101] Dr. Langer thought that that figure might have been an exaggeration until he started to test his own patients and came to the conclusion that not only was Dr. Barnes probably correct, but he may well have underestimated the true extent of the condition.

It would be reasonable to suggest that a similar percentage of the British population might also have compromised states of health, as both nations have similar diets of heavily processed foods.

A reduced body temperature is almost certainly the product of long-term poor nutrition. A poor diet sustained over many years can impair the health of a person so that the glands responsible for well-being function less efficiently than they should. When such denatured nutrition impairs the endocrine glands and the function of the thyroid system is interfered with, the result will mean reduced body temperature and all that goes with such a condition…

An example of how improved nutrition can turn around someone with reduced thyroid function, and therefore low body temperature, comes from Janet Pleshette's *Cures That Work*.[102] In it there is an interview with a patient with severe hypothyroidism who was given months to live unless she took daily doses of thyroid tablets.

Being an advocate of Nature Cure and a founder member of Tyringham Nature Cure Clinic in England, she decided that she didn't want to live for the rest of her life on drugs and went to the clinic instead. Her severely bloated appearance was such that the staff at the clinic were reluctant to take her in, but did so eventually. After a week, with no improvement, she was about to leave when she bumped into a Sri Lankan doctor at the clinic who asked if he could take on her case. Her appearance alerted him to the fact that she was hypothyroid and he was confident he could turn her health around.

The doctor gave her acupuncture and advised her to change to a natural diet of fruits and vegetables. She was also instructed to eliminate all dairy products. It wasn't long before her symptoms abated, her appearance changed and her health returned – all by application of a natural approach and without thyroid tablets. After several months she was back to being completely normal, much to the astonishment of her own G.P.

The natural diet of the Gerson Therapy has also restored to health many patients who had symptoms of reduced thyroid activity. Charlotte Gerson, the daughter of Dr. Max Gerson, has kindly allowed me to quote one such case. Elizabeth B., suffered from a number of symptoms including hypothyroidism. She had been put on several drugs, to no avail. She had multiple allergies, but after a slow but steady improvement on the Gerson Therapy she recovered her health completely. Another way of reading this is that improved nutrition returned her body temperature to normal – as was evidenced by her return to health.

Further insight

When I delved further into the link between body temperature and illness, more and more information appeared, which, on its own, did not mean much, but when added to other parts of the jigsaw, gave a wonderful insight into just what was happening in the food allergic patient.

I have been able to find that hyperactivity, a familiar symptom linked to food/chemical allergies, and other neurological problems, can be the result of pinworm (*Enterobius vermicularis*) infestation.[103] Not everyone with pinworm infection however develops such problems, and the more common symptom caused by these creatures resembling three-quarter inch threads is anal itching. But the fact that the classic food allergy condition of hyperactivity is being linked at all with a parasite is further evidence of the almost-certain underestimation of the true extent to which micro-organisms are causing us illness.

Another temperature 'surprise'

As I delved even further, although I was focussing really on the conditions known to have a food allergy connection, other surprises awaited. One of the exciting 'discoveries' I made was in the field of electro-physiology.

Harking back to when I was a teenager, when I was foolishly experimenting with street drugs such as purple hearts, I recalled the vastly improved powers of concentration that I would experience when under the influence of these tablets. As the general improvement, not only in my concentration span, but wellbeing, was so dramatic, it was probably no wonder that I should have become addicted.

One of the approaches I considered, when looking for the cause of my own illness, was to find out just exactly what the mechanism was behind the actions of amphetamines such as 'purple hearts'. If I could find out what they did in my body, therein would lie a clue to the overall illness.

Incidentally, the accepted treatment for many children with ADD – that is Attention Deficit Disorder, where children suffer from hyperactivity and reduced attention span – has been amphetamines! Whilst these would certainly improve the lot of the child, and be a grateful crutch to a harassed mother, drugs can only ever be short-lasting support. They will never remove the cause.

I had looked into the pharmaceutical effects of amphetamines before, but had never been able to link their effects on the neurotransmitters in the brain to anything significant, until this body temperature and parasite discovery, when things started to look a whole lot clearer.

During my research I came across the wonderful surprise that temperature was involved in the elusive wellbeing afford by the amphetamines! It transpired that the mechanism behind amphetamines includes the 'speeding-up' of neurotransmitters in the brain. These are electrical signals that fire from one neuron in the brain to the next, jumping gaps called synapses.

A slowing down of these electrical firings can result in poor cerebral performance, and, conversely, if such activity is speeded up, alertness and wellbeing can result. It took some time before I connected with the fact that body temperature plays an important part in neuronal activity!

Electro-physiologists specialise in the study of electrical activity that naturally occurs within the body, the most marked area of such activity being in the brain, where the vast cerebral arterial network and the infinite number of electrical connections defy any attempts to rationalise their patterns.

Scientists discovered that neurons are temperature-sensitive, or 'thermo-sensitive'.[104] The neurotransmitters respond to changes in temperature with significant changes in their firing rates. It is known that the firing rates of neurotransmitters increase when the temperature is higher and this activity reduces when the temperature drops.

The phenomenon of the 'endorphin high' that is talked about in exercise circles is another indicator of how body temperature can play a part in wellbeing. Exercise is known to increase core body temperature!

This brief look into the pharmacological action of amphetamines served an important purpose for me. I could now make several connections, between my poor attention span when younger, its huge improvement when on amphetamines, the improved feeling of wellbeing I had when taking them, my known later reduced body temperature and subsequent poor health with food allergies and, behind all of this, the new-found link to body temperature.

Arthritis as a weather forecaster?

It has long been part of folklore that elderly people can 'predict' the onset of an attack of arthritis by a change in the weather. Often they will say that its going to rain when they feel a twinge of their condition.

We know that arthritis is directly linked with food allergies. We now see that parasites are connected to the food allergy response. And we know these parasites are temperature-sensitive. Does this provide a firm basis for the apparent ability to 'forecast' an attack of arthritis?

Psychic healing?

Although I am certainly not advocating psychic healing, one wonders if the 'intense heat' at the site of the symptom many people refer to, might have some basis in truth, in that the healer is able to somehow pass his heat into someone who was less 'thermally endowed' so to speak, thus temporarily inactivating any problem parasites?

13.

The Food Allergy Reaction: 'Simple' Obstruction?

The entire mechanism behind 'masked food allergy', which is really any illness that can be shown to have a dietary link to symptoms, is still not fully known. My view, having satisfied myself that parasites are linked to the 'food allergic' reaction or indeed to any illness that has a food implication, is that there is 'simple' blockage or obstruction to the blood flow or, in the case of breathing problems, the airways, at the site of the symptom.

It is quite clear also that if 1 billion people around the planet have the parasite *Ascaris lumbricoides* within them, then that parasite, for one, has been totally successful in avoiding all our immunological defences.[105]

Whilst most micro-organisms are destroyed by our defence barriers such as the sweat and sebum of our skin; the anti-microbial products in our saliva and tears; the hairs and mucous membranes in our nose; the mucous secretions from our respiratory tract, and our gastric juices, it is clear that many parasites, for example protozoa and helminths, can successfully enter – and flourish for decades – in our system. Protozoan parasites, for example, are transmitted in cyst form, a sac-like structure that protects the organism from defences such as gastric secretions.[106]

Having breached our defences, what part do they play in illness, especially the one we refer to as food allergy? We must recognise that during the acute response to an incoming food, the patient will experience a reduced blood flow at the site of the symptom, or the closing of the lumen of the alveoli in the case of breathing trouble such as asthma.[107, 108]

The reduction in blood flow – the hypoperfusion – will have come about through some response by the parasite to the incoming food/chemical allergen. It is severely tempting to suggest it is simply a blockage in the blood flow. It would make eminent sense to offer the hypothesis that, once these organisms, at the site of the symptom, sense the 'taint' or 'signature' of the substance entering the system, they respond in some fashion that produces blockage.

The fact that someone merely has to inhale an allergenic substance in order to undergo a reaction clearly demonstrates that the allergen does not have to enter the body by the gastrointestinal tract. There is also the phenomenon of someone holding a glass jar with an allergenic food inside it, and the patient reacting to the substance inside the glass! A process is involved in these allergic responses that is simply beyond our comprehension.

All living things vibrate. All living things give out a frequency. All living things resonate. We are also electrical beings. We all have electric activity surging through our bodies. We also emit electrical signals. Dr. Hulda Clark uses these frequencies to identify the presence of parasites.

Could the cheese in the glass jar, for example, be emitting signals that 'meet' or 'clash' with the signals of electrical activity emanating from our bodies, such trigger then coursing through the watery medium that is our body, 'tainting' our blood with that substance and their presence being sensed by these primitive organisms?

The mechanism involved could be a form of positive chemotaxis, whereby the parasite recognises a substance by mere chemical 'taint' of the bloodstream, and responds accordingly. Such responses by parasites to chemical stimuli are known in parasite physiology and can play an essential part in the parasite locating an appropriate host.

For example, a monogenean parasite of European marine flatfish, *Entobdella soleae,* is able to locate its preferred host (sole) by chemical recognition of the fish skin.[109] Perhaps this unique sensory skill plays no small part in what we know as simple food/chemical allergy responses.

You only have to release a tiny droplet of ink into a bowl of water to see how readily and comprehensively it is disseminated through the entire water. Perhaps a similar mechanism based on electrical frequencies exists.

However it works, those of us who have experienced bizarre 'allergic' responses merely by inhaling a substance, know only too well that it can happen.

Is the parasite's nutrition the key to the allergic response?

If we can uncover what the nutrition of the micro-organism is, perhaps therein would lie the clue to the food allergic response.

If a sufferer can experience a migraine on eating a sausage roll, and experience exactly the same migraine on inhaling perfume as he walks past the perfume counter in a department store, then there has to be some common denominator. But no-one has been able to work out exactly what that could be.

Now that we know micro-organisms are involved in the allergic response, perhaps their diet is what we should be looking at to see what sets them off.

Whilst very little is known about the physiological requirements of these creatures, perhaps recent work by marine geologists has supplied us with a vital clue to this mystery. Scientists studying underwater volcanoes have been raising lava chimneys from deep in the ocean in order to study these structures. What they discovered was that there was a multitude of microbial life within these formations and that they lived and thrived on the gases produced by such volcanic activity!

In the migraine sufferer, as the sausage roll would result in metabolic gases being spread throughout the bloodstream by diffusion, then it could be these chemical gases that would be sensed by the micro-organisms telling them food has arrived, triggering off their activity. So too could the inhalation of a perfume – an aeroallergen – similarly produce gases in the blood. It is these chemical gases that seem the certain common denominator.

Which neatly returns me to the 1970s when I first found out I was allergic in Rome. They used sniff testing on me. They didn't know how the sniff tests worked, they just knew that they did. Now 30 years on, I have found out what was surely happening then: we were providing the parasites with a meal of gases which produced activity on their part.

But once these micro-organisms sense the incoming food (the gases), what occurs next? Whether it is a food or an inhaled substance, what occurs to bring about the allergic symptom? As there is an interference in blood flow, it seems logical to assume there might be simple blockage.

The 'simple' blockage theory is as good as any. But do the parasites engorge themselves with blood at the sense of the mere 'taint' of the blood by a particular incoming allergen? Does this simple engorgement by perhaps a huge number of tiny organisms bring about sufficient occlusion in a small arteriole, too fast for any collateral circulation to develop, and therefore produce such hypoperfusion? Or do these micro-organisms secrete a substance in response to such incoming food or chemical, producing inflammation, which closes off the blood supply in that area?

The inflammation hypothesis isn't so appealing, as these reactions often disappear entirely within an hour and inflammation is unlikely to do that.

What about change of activity? Upon sensing the incoming allergen, these parasites may thrash about, in whatever way they can, perhaps in a similar fashion to small birds in a nest all straining their necks and preparing themselves for a feeding frenzy when they sense the mother returning with food. Could a similar frenzy of activity occur when parasites sense the 'signature' in the blood of the incoming allergenic agent? Would that be enough to bring about the activity to produce reduced blood flow?

If that were the case, it would incur inflammation, and as I have said, inflammation seems unlikely as the reaction often wears off too quickly to support that hypothesis.

I favour mere engorgement, mere change in shape, creating a 'simple' mechanical blockage or obstruction of blood flow.

There is nothing 'simple' about 'simple' blockage. Blockage of the blood flow to the heart for example can bring about an end to your entire life. Simple blockage anywhere in the body will result in symptoms of pain or distress of some sort. I think that the simple blockage hypothesis will prove in time to be far more common than hitherto considered.

And if the reader thinks that "simple blockage" anywhere in the body may be too lowly an explanation for a chronic illness that has baffled doctors for years, let me introduce a quote from *Modern Parasitology* which gives support to that very possibility:

> Both lymphatic and ocular filariasis are accompanied by gross pathological changes, elephantiasis and blindness, but it is not clear if these have any immunological basis and current opinion favours simple obstruction.[110]

Note that it says 'current opinion'. It appears that they have been so in the dark, despite all the books on the subject of parasitology and in particular filariasis, that only, in 1999, did they realise that simple blockage held the key to the illness.

Here are some more offerings to suggest simple blockage may play a part: From *Microbial and Parasite Infection*:

> Mechanical blockage can be a major component of the diseases caused by some parasites – e.g. obstruction of the gut lumen by large numbers of Ascaris or by smaller numbers of tapeworms; or obstruction of intestinal absorption by large numbers of Giardia covering the wall of the small intestine.[111]

From *Modern Parasitology* (p40), discussing the parasite *Schistosome haematobium*:

> Granulomatous reactions, and later fibrosis and calcification, induce a wide range of pathological manifestations including haematuria and dysuria, hyperplasia of the bladder lining which can progress to bladder cancer, partial blockage of the ureters and secondary damage to the kidneys.[112]

Finally the most important quote in *Modern Parasitology*, as far as I am concerned, the one that serves to confirm my theory that simple blockage plays a major part in the food allergic illness, given that we know there is a reduced blood flow during a reaction, is reproduced here:

Pairs of adult worms produce eggs which are laid into the lumina of the venules in which they live. There is no direct, non-pathological route by which these eggs can reach the outside world from this location. In fact, most schistosome eggs possess a sharp shell spine which helps to provide a means of escape. Spines lodge in the intima of the venule and impede the movement of eggs by blood flow. Small blood vessels packed with eggs may rupture, enabling them to move into surrounding connective tissue.[113]

Here we have confirmation that;

(i)   parasites can indeed lodge, live in, and reproduce in, blood vessel walls.
(ii) they are capable of impeding the flow of blood by their presence.
(iii) blood vessels can be 'packed' with eggs so severely that the vessel can rupture.

It is therefore quite clear to my mind that the 'food allergic' reaction is 'simple' blockage in a blood vessel at the site of the symptom, brought about by parasitic activity in that blood vessel.

14.

Raise Your
Body Temperature Naturally

A subnormal body temperature and poor health go hand in hand. The lowered temperature is indicative of lowered vitality, which can leave us open to all manner of illness, including infestation by predatory micro-organisms. In the plant kingdom, it is those plants with reduced vitality that are attacked by parasites. It is the same, it seems, in human beings.

Many health problems can be caused by low body temperature but this connection between the patient's problems and his core body temperature is regularly missed by doctors. Part of the reason why it can be overlooked is because hospital blood tests for thyroid function often return as normal when in fact the patient might well have disturbed thyroid activity. The patient may have a sub-clinical thyroid system dysfunction, one that is not full-blown, and the blood tests simply do not pick this up.

The reason such blood tests can be unreliable is that they gauge glandular function by measuring levels of thyroid hormones in the *bloodstream*. But the thyroid hormones have their action in the cells of the body at the nuclear membrane receptors and there is no method of accurately measuring such intracellular activity.

The test results might well show a satisfactory level of the thyroid hormone T4 and even TSH (thyroid stimulating hormone) but the patient could still have a problem in converting the T4 hormone to the more active T3 hormone. How well this conversion takes place will determine the efficiency of his or her thyroid system function.

Blood tests can be useful insofar as extremely low blood values can be indicative of extremely low body temperature, and extremely high blood values can indicate extremely high body temperature. But when the results are not so extreme, the picture becomes more blurred.

Some patients with reduced thyroid functioning benefit from added thyroid supplementation in the form of thyroxine (T4). However an unknown number of patients will have problems converting T4 to T3 (tri-iodothyronine), the more active hormone. These patients might well get little or no benefit from such T4 therapy and falsely therefore consider their thyroid function normal.

In the long run, adding a tablet to the body of someone with long-term health problems merely provides a crutch. Helpful though it may be to some patients, the real answer will only ever be found when the *cause* of the dysfunctioning thyroid system is addressed.

I show in this book that body temperature can rise when eating a *natural* diet. We have, therefore, found the cause of the low body temperature: the patient's previous diet!

Long term poor diet choice, sometimes over decades, will mean that the tissues and organs of the body have been deprived of the multitude of nutrients that Nature intended. The 'correction' of such long term impairment will not be addressed by a simple tablet or two. The patient might get relief from his symptoms for a while by taking a thyroid tablet, but for his health to be fully and permanently restored, the *cause* of the low body temperature, his former diet, has to be removed.

Let us imagine, for a moment, an anthropoid ape, the animal closest in appearance and physiological make-up to man. That animal was intended, in nature, to eat any number of juicy fruits and occasionally plants, for its entire lifespan. We are aware that that animal will develop the immensely powerful structure typical of its species. The closeness of the anthropoid ape's make-up to the human's is astonishing (see Chapter 23, *What Man Should Eat*).

The ape is not a carnivore, nor an omnivore; it is a fruitarian or herbivore. The huge muscular frame will come from fruits and plants, not the protein of meat. Whilst humans seem to think that they need to eat meat (protein) in order to develop muscles, Nature is telling us that this is not the case at all.

Let us now view what might happen if an ape, very similar to man, were to eat a sustained unnatural diet.

Let us start with a baby ape and deprive it of the nutrition that is correct for its species. Instead, we will feed it on artificial foods such as those we might give a human baby and child: tinned foods, artificial baby milk, processed foods, foods and drinks grossly over-heated and therefore enzyme-less, colas, chocolate bars, and other abominations of nutrition that modern humans seem to consider as perfectly normal.

Now let us continue feeding that ape with this artificial and unnatural diet, not just for ten days, but for, say, thirty years. Compared to his fellow 30-year-old companion ape, who is fed the nutrition Nature intended him, our example will be deprived of a lifetime of natural foods.

As body organs will have been denied the natural foods that should gone into them in order to build and sustain health, it is inevitable that the thirty-year-old ape fed artificially will have compromised health compared to his naturally-fed friend.

If the artificially-fed animal now has a malfunctioning thyroid gland, no single tablet of thyroxine can reasonably be expected to take the place of thirty years of fruits and restore health to tissues and organs deficient in any number of nutritional elements which would naturally have been provided.

The thyroid gland will function most sweetly when all other parts are working synergistically with it. If all parts of the body have been deprived correct nutrition, then all manner of dysfunctions will have taken place, and an unnatural state of disorganised atrophy will exist.

The only correct method of restoring health to that animal, in compliance with the laws of Nature, would be to correct its nutrition and wait to see the results. It may be too late, after 30 years, but that is the only option. At the very least, partial recovery will surely take place.

All physiological requirements and processes have to be in tune and working together synergistically – like an orchestra – in order to achieve the *natural* climb in vitality, in body temperature, to restore health. No one single tablet can achieve all that on a permanent basis.

It is the same in humans. Anyone with a reduced body temperature or underactive thyroid gland requires more than a simple thyroid tablet. He or she will need to have their diet corrected to as near a natural one as possible and be able to sustain it, before results can be expected. There is no short cut.

We know from our experience and work in nutrition that reduced vitality (and body temperature) is in the first place down to what one inherits at birth; to this we have to add whatever diet we choose to pursue.

That correction of diet can restore health, we know. Even doctors, untrained in the link between natural diet and healing, could not fault the logic behind the concept that improved nutrition is good for you.

Sustained attempts at an intensively-applied natural diet, either in Nature Cure establishments, or from records of patients who have undergone the Gerson Therapy, show that recovery from all manner of ill health is possible.

Let us go back to our apes. If you were presented with the two apes, and told that the supremely healthy one was fed all the fruits and plants it wanted, while the other specimen, with all manner of symptoms such as poor fur, bad teeth, poor skeletal formation, constant fatigue, disinterest in his surroundings, and perhaps to round it off, irritability, was fed exclusively on chocolate bars and fizzy drinks, what would seem the logical thing to do to try to bring health to the latter?

Surely we would, as one, shout that it should be fed a natural diet. Give it the fruits it was intended to eat, just like its healthy companion. Yet we seem to miss this simple solution if we are presented with a similar situation involving humans!

Going back to the snake in the vet analogy, any vet would instruct you to start feeding the ill snake its natural diet if you were to admit that you were feeding it white-bread sandwiches.

Man was not intended to eat highly processed, highly heated foods. Look at Chapter 23 (*How Man Should Eat*), for an indication of what was intended before we became too clever at food adulteration and processing for our own good.

Man can recover from all manner of ills IF he can prise himself away from the highly unnatural and, more importantly, extremely addictive diet that he will have been brought up on. Our modern society is fed wrongly and unnaturally. It takes considerable determination and guts to change – and stick to – a natural diet of virtually all fruits and vegetables, soups, and some cereals.

But those who do, and there are many, have reported absolutely stunning turnarounds in health. It should be expected too. The ape should expect improved health. The snake should be expected to feel the benefit of having his unnatural diet removed. And so should man.

To raise the body temperature from subnormal to a naturally high one is eminently achievable by diet alone. Filling your diet now with as much fruit as possible can go a long way to reversing the actual cause of the reduced core temperature in the first place.

15.

Food Allergies and their Symptoms

Whilst many readers will be familiar with the food allergy syndrome and all its associated disorders, many more will not. Please therefore forgive me if I am preaching to the converted!

David was a successful construction engineer with his own thriving company. He drove a luxury car and money was no object. He had a good family life and should have been very happy. But David suffered from depression.

His doctor was a personal friend of the family and would often be invited to David's house for dinner. However close the doctor was to the family, he could offer David no further help beyond the obligatory tranquillisers and anti-depressants. This he had done regularly for the ten years David had been ill. Despite this well-meaning pharmacological attention, David's condition did not improve.

When David came to me for help, I gave him instructions to stick to a restricted diet for a number of days to see how he felt. After five days David returned, stating he was feeling much happier than he had for many a long year.

Having previously received a sample list of David's usual diet by post, I had prepared some ten test food items which I felt might well be problem foods for him. As each test – by the sub-lingual (under the tongue) challenge method – took about 8 minutes, I could not afford the time to carry out more tests per visit and he was given advice on how to test himself for further foods when he got home.

David showed no reaction whatsoever to the first nine food tests. On the tenth and final one (he did not know it was to be the last test) his face displayed great anxiety, whilst he used both hands to grip the edge of my desk. Panicking, he said 'You'll have to do something about this, I feel terrible.' I had ready a remedy – an almost homoeopathically–diluted version of the very substance that had produced this major reaction. Introducing a drop under his tongue immediately caused a reduction in the severity. By further reducing the strength of the substance, I was able to switch his reaction off entirely.

David was delighted. For the first time in ten years he had something by which to control his debilitating illness without the use of drugs. He had found a trigger for this most distressing of conditions. The very finding of such a dietary trigger in itself removed the suggestion that the condition was of a mental or psychiatric nature; at last he knew it to be physical.

Mike was 28, a former keen amateur footballer who had for the last three years suffered inexplicable bouts of sheer fatigue. Every movement was an effort and he spent virtually all day either in bed or lying on the sofa watching television. His mother called him the classic 'couch potato', but both she and Mike knew there was something wrong, as he had previously always been extremely energetic. He had given up his beloved football because he could not find the energy to do the necessary training, and, of course, he knew he was not entirely well.

His doctor could find no obvious reason for Mike's condition but referred him to hospital for blood tests. All were negative and it was ever so kindly suggested that perhaps he was imagining it! Mike had tried all sorts of over-the-counter pick-me-ups in an effort to regain his former energy. Some worked briefly but none truly addressed the cause.

When I saw the daily diet that he had written down for me, I could see that there was vast room for improvement in the actual nutritional status, besides the strong possibility that some of his food choices were allergenic to him. Virtually everything he ate was either deficient, packaged or tinned. When it wasn't packaged or tinned it was confectionery. And he smoked 25 cigarettes a day.

When I explained that there was room for improvement in his diet, he said he couldn't fathom why his diet should be at fault as the diet he had now was exactly the same as when he was full of energy and playing football. I had to explain that this was like a cancer patient in an iron lung asking how he could possibly be in this condition due to cigarettes, when 20 years ago he smoked the same number as he did now and didn't have any health problems!

After ten days on fruits only, he came back reporting a huge change in his energy levels. When I tested him for white bread, he was virtually rooted to his seat; he also recognised that a 'mental dullness' that he had complained of had returned. Mike went away with information that had not been available to him elsewhere. He was far happier now that he had something tangible to explain away his 'unexplained' fatigue to his mother and his friends.

Sandra, a 38-year-old, came to me with depression and nervousness that had made her life a misery for years. After following a restricted diet for several days she returned to my office for testing. All the tests were blind, in that she did not know what items were being tested, either by taste or by the colour of the liquid. Any suggestion or psychological influence could therefore be discounted.

She reacted to only one food item amongst the ten being tested: Granny Smith's apples! On introduction of the liquefied food, she suffered an instant and severe bout of depression. Thankfully I was able to introduce an antidote that switched off the reaction.

Naturally she was delighted, as she had for the first time found a reason behind her seemingly unexplained illness. A national newspaper wanted to write a story about her case and how such a simple thing as a Granny Smith's apple could cause depression. Though Sandra was happy enough to confirm the story, she was adamant that she would not be photographed for a newspaper, so it was dropped.

I give you the above examples to show that ordinary, everyday illnesses such as fatigue, depression or nervousness, can have a dietary link, without your doctor ever being aware food can be a factor in the condition. Similarly, many other physical and mental disorders can have a food connection.

We who have made the jump to recognising that certain foods can trigger our symptoms are fortunate, but there are untold numbers of people who have still not been able to link their symptoms to their diets, despite much publicity about the phenomenon in the media over the last few decades.

Responsibility for general lack of awareness of the condition partly rests with your average G.P., who still doesn't know the techniques required to identify offending foods. It is often the case that the G.P. simply doesn't want to accept such a seemingly 'simple' explanation for conditions that have baffled him and his peers. Because it wasn't part of his teaching at medical school, he either does not believe in the condition or is resistant to the very concept.

Doctors do not get any training in the food allergy connection to common health disorders at medical school; but that does not mean that the patient himself cannot take a degree of control over his own condition.

The food allergic patient might appear to be obsessed with his or her diet; and to be fair, no one can blame him. After all, if every time you passed a cocker spaniel in the street you developed an excruciating pain in your knees, then no-one would blame you for being obsessed with cocker spaniels... The cocker spaniel in this case is the foods we put into our mouths.

It is even more understandable that many food allergics become over-obsessed with their diet if and when many become 'universal reactors', that is they get symptoms after eating or drinking practically everything. The patient who has made the food connection to his symptoms – the food allergic sufferer – is still, even today, in a tiny minority group. He or she often feels totally alone, having little or no contact with other knowledgeable sufferers, whilst being surrounded by family and friends who often will consider him or her a food crank, or 'nut'.

However, once someone has made the dramatic (and it unquestionably is dramatic) discovery that their long-hated symptoms can be switched on by taking in foods they have been consuming since childhood with seeming impunity, then their life suddenly gains a degree of stability that was long lacking.

Often food allergies are referred to by other writers as food 'intolerances' or food 'hypersensitivities'. It should be noted that whilst organic foods can themselves bring about a reaction, chemical components or adulterants in foods can also provoke a response, so food allergy, intolerance, or hypersensitivity are merely umbrella descriptions covering the dietary link to illness. Common usage dictates we keep to food 'allergy' however.

A milestone discovery

Once you have identified foods which can 'bring on' your symptoms, you will have passed a major milestone in your life. There can be no turning back once the discovery is made. You will become one of a growing band of aware patients who will have, for the first time, accessed a definite trigger which can bring on an acute attack of their hated symptoms.

The only 'drawback' to being a diet-aware person is that you may well be unfairly accused of falling into the 'obsessed with your diet' category. But you will be forever grateful for having made such a discovery, because it will not only help you in your entire future life, but you will be provided with a simple tool which you can put to great use with your entire family's future health.

Whoever makes the discovery of a link between symptoms and diet will see before them the prospect of release from a lifetime of unnecessary suffering. The food allergy concept needs no external salesman to press home the point; the patient will see for himself and experience within his own body the return of symptoms on consuming culprit foods. There can be no better salesman than that.

This relatively recent finding – made over the last 30 or so years - that many ordinary health problems can be diet-linked has led countless people around the world to recognise that they do indeed have these food allergies. The huge band of patients, alert to the connection their doctors have missed, is increasing all the time.

The majority of us in the 'civilised' world have these food 'allergies'. Using this book, it will be relatively easy to identify a dietary connection to your health if, after eating a suspect food, you watch as the unmistakeable symptoms appear over and over again. The experiments you will make will be 'reproducible' – that is you will be able to make the connection (food and symptom) time after time. This is what orthodox medicine insists should be the case to prove something is valid. 'Reproducibility' is a 'scientific' factor in assessing the validity of a concept. There are few areas where the reproducibility factor comes over louder or clearer than in the food allergy condition, yet orthodox medicine still has difficulty in accepting it.

It is unquestionably a comfort to many patients to have some degree of control over their condition, and without the need for drugs. It is more often than not the case that their doctor, unaware of the food connection, will merely dish out a pharmaceutical preparation – a prescribed drug – in an attempt to minimise the actual symptoms. Fine though that may have been up to a point, such drug taking merely temporarily influences the course of the condition and does nothing to find the actual cause of the disorder. Furthermore, no one knows for sure what long term consequences there will be on the patient's overall health as a result of this often indiscriminate use of commonly-prescribed drugs. But using this book, mere dietary change can reduce your symptoms, without the use of drugs.

The conditions linked to food allergies

Because of the vast number of ordinary conditions linked to food allergies, many doctors have difficulty in accepting the very existence of the syndrome.

The food allergy claim that so many seemingly separate conditions can be brought on by eating foods or consuming drinks to which the patient may have a 'hidden' allergy is a valid credibility-reducing factor.

The very length of the following list of apparently disparate disorders adds to the disbelief or even incredulity. The sheer number of diverse conditions claimed to be the result of eating 'ordinary' foods almost ensures the syndrome is relegated to the shelf of the charlatan or put into the category of the quacks and their bottles of 'Elixir of Youth'. But the undeniable fact – to which hundreds of thousands of people can testify – is that virtually any condition can indeed be triggered by simply consuming everyday foods or drinks.

The far deeper truth about the food allergy position is that virtually *everyone* with the undermentioned conditions will have a dietary link to their illness. It is only the relatively few patients who proceed down the line of proper dietary investigation who discover this fact. If everyone with such illnesses properly examined their diets, then the number of people with 'food allergy' in the world would explode overnight beyond recognition!

SYMPTOMS OF FOOD/CHEMICAL ALLERGY

Table 1

Some Symptoms or Conditions Found to be Caused
by Foods, Drinks or Chemical Allergy

I Appearance and skin
acne
canker sores
dark circles under eyes
dermatitis
eczema
hives
itching
pale colour not due to anaemia
psoriasis
skin reddening.

II Headache
various kinds including migraine

III Eye Conditions
conjunctivitis
eye pain
periods of blurred vision
sensitivity to light
tearing
temporary refractive changes

IV Ear Conditions
hearing loss
infections
inflammations
Meniere's syndrome
noises in the ear
repeated ear trouble

V Cardiovascular
angina
high blood pressure
irregular heartbeat
low blood pressure
rapid pulse

VI Gastrointestinal
constipation
diarrhoea
gall bladder pains
wind
gastric ulcer
gastro-intestinal bleeding
heartburn
haemorrhoids
indigestion
mucous colitis
nausea
nervous stomach
pains or cramps
spastic colon
vomiting

VII Respiratory
asthma
chronic rhinitis
coughing
frequent 'colds'
hay fever

VII Respiratory (continued)
mouth breathing
nosebleeds
postnasal discharge
sinusitis
stuffy nose
wheezing

VIII Urological
bedwetting
frequent night urination
frequent urination
painful or difficult urination

IX Muscular-skeletal
arthritis
joint pains
muscle cramps
muscle aches and pains
muscle spasms
muscle weakness

X Mental-behavioural
anxiety
delusions
depression (including psychotic)
dizzy spells
drowsiness
epilepsy
floating sensations
general fatigue

X Mental-behavioural (continues)
hallucinations
hyperactivity
insomnia
irritability
learning disorders
minimal brain dysfunction
nervousness
periods of confusion
phobias
poor concentration
poor memory
poor muscle coordination
restlessness
schizophrenia
sleeps at inappropriate times
sleeps too little
sleeps too much
tension-fatigue syndrome
unsteadiness

XI Other
abnormal body odour
diabetes
excessive sweating
general weakness
hypoglycaemia
night-sweating
overweight
underweight
virus infections

The above list is reproduced from *How to Control Your Allergies.*[120]

At first glance, it is understandable why many doctors baulk at such a wide spread of symptoms being put down to food allergies; but the knowledge that blood flow is interfered with should serve to explain.

16.

How to Test for Food Allergies

One of the most accurate methods of testing for food and chemical allergies is by monitoring your pulse. Watch for a speeding up or slowing down after eating, in conjunction with any change in your symptoms.

Hospital skin tests for masked food allergies have been shown to be notoriously unreliable indicators of true masked food allergy. They may well show up some reactions to foods or other substances, but that is no proof that such 'allergies' play any part in the patient's actual symptoms. Indeed, more often than not, they don't.

Such tests therefore serve no real purpose other than to further confuse the patient looking for a diet link to his symptoms. They can be a real backward step in the patient's attempt to recover from his illness. The false information provided will put him on an entirely wrong track that he might well stay on for the rest of his life – unless he learns new methods of testing.

Your pulse

Your pulse should be at its lowest reading first thing in the morning, before you get out of bed. However, if you indulged in a heavy meal the night before, full of allergenic foods, your morning's pulse reading might still be affected. This is a phenomenon of which you will have to be aware during your testing.

Your aim is to arrive at your normal lowest pulse reading. This may take a few days to achieve, as you remove, one by one, the allergenic foods from your diet. But once your meals are free from such foods, only then should your morning reading show your true, minimum pulse rate.

If your morning pulse rate is not the lowest reading of the day, and if this carries on during the days of testing, suspect something in your house. Perhaps you may have an unsuspected 'allergy' to the gas fire in your lounge or bedroom. If this is so, your pulse rate can be influenced by it. Even a new carpet or the bedding itself may be suspect.

Be aware that seemingly innocuous items like fresh newsprint, soap, or even toothpaste can have a bearing on your pulse if you are susceptible to them.

Once your lowest pulse rate is established, by daily attention to your allergens (substances to which you are allergic), there are certain features of food and chemical allergies that can be accurately applied and used as a guide to assess your progress. These are:

(1) From your lowest pulse reading of the day to your highest should not exceed 16 beats – assuming freedom from fever, sunburn, strenuous exercise or drugs.

(2) Your pulse reading should differ little when sitting or standing. If it does this indicates existing allergic tension.

(3) Whilst psychological or emotional stress may affect the pulse, repeated reaction to a direct food challenge indicates an allergy.

(4) A rested pulse reading above 84 indicates allergy – even in children.

The textbook 'average' pulse is 72, but everybody has their own individual normal rate. You will be able to ascertain your own normal average pulse as your food testing progresses and allergenic foods or drinks are eliminated

How to take your pulse

Turn your left hand over, so that it is palm up. Take the first two fingers of your right hand and place them on the centre of your left wrist, about an inch up from where the hand joins the wrist. Now move the fingers to halfway between where your fingers presently are sitting and the outer (left) edge of the wrist. There is a sort of 'gulley' and your pulse is in there. There is no need for heavy pressure; a light touch is all that is required to feel the pulse. The more you practise taking it, the easier it will become. You will soon find yourself taking it many times a day simply out of ongoing curiosity, and it will become second nature.

For food allergy testing purposes it is important that you take the count for a full 60 seconds and not for 15 seconds and then multiply it by 4, or for 30 seconds then multiply it by 2, as nurses may do. That is because a mere few beats difference, which may be hidden by such shortcuts, can make all the difference between identifying a safe or an unsafe substance.

On the day you decide to start your food tests, take your pulse before you get out of bed. The morning reading should get lower as the days progress and as you discover, then remove the culprit foods, etc. from your diet. It is essential that you keep a food diary, writing down everything you eat and drink and at what time, along with your pulse readings.

Make three columns in your food diary with these headings:

(1) Safe Foods (2) Forbidden Foods (3) Under Suspicion

Test your meals by taking your pulse just before eating, then again three more times after each meal, each reading being half an hour apart. Write down your pulse readings.

If your pulse accelerates or slows down by eight or more beats (per full minute) after eating, then that food must go in the 'Forbidden Foods' column. Your pulse will not be greatly affected by ordinary physical activity, so it is not essential to sit still like a dummy for the entire 90 minutes awaiting the pulse readings! However, for the three readings during testing it is always best to sit down for a few minutes prior to pulse-taking, so as to ensure an unconfused reading.

After a few days some sort of pattern will emerge and you will be able to spot the meals which influenced your pulse. However, you may not know which of the ingredients within any meal caused the pulse to be affected.

The reason for testing entire meals for a few days is to get you into the way of testing and at the same time to give you a recognisable pattern of pulse-influencing mealtimes which will serve to prove to you that you do indeed have food allergies.

You can now choose your day on which to isolate and test individual foods. That day should start, as usual, with pulse-taking – in bed.

The second pulse reading will be taken when you are seated, just before your first meal. You should eat an average-sized portion of a regularly consumed food, say, potatoes. Do not add anything such as butter or pepper, as you are testing only the actual food.

Take your pulse again 30 minutes after eating the food, then again a further 30 minutes later, and finally again 30 minutes on. To summarise:

(i)   Take your pulse before the meal, then:
(ii) 30 minutes after eating
(iii) 60 minutes after eating
(iv) 90 minutes after eating

If your pulse moves, up or down, 8 or more beats per minute from the pre-meal reading, allergy is indicated. If you get any symptoms, say headache or dizziness, even without a pulse change, this can still be indicative of food allergy, and that particular food should go in the 'Under Suspicion' column, to be tested again at a later date to see if the same symptoms re-appear. This re-testing of foods that may not influence the pulse but which may bring on any symptom, should only be carried out FIVE DAYS after the first test.

If, after the 90 minutes have passed, your pulse has not changed and no symptoms have occurred, that food can be put in the 'Safe Foods' column and you may start your next food test immediately. However, if your pulse does change, or if any symptoms should appear, you must wait both until your pulse returns to the pre-test reading and the symptoms have worn off before starting your next food test.

A typical pulse diary – when testing foods – would look something like this:

Pulse Readings

Time	Food	Before Food	After 30 mins	After 60 mins	After 90 mins
12:00 noon	GRAPES	68	68	68	68
1.30 pm	BANANAS	68	83	87	74

On the above test, grapes – if you did not get any symptoms during the test – have proven to be safe. But the bananas caused the pulse to jump more than 8 beats; it jumped 15 at its highest, so bananas would be put in the Forbidden Foods column, whether or not you experienced any symptoms during the test.

You should wait until your pulse returns to 68 after the banana test – and any symptoms have gone – before proceeding to the next test.

The symptoms that may occur can be many and varied, and all too often come as a complete surprise to the tester. Long standing complaints which may be tolerable before a meal, may become quite severe afterwards and it is this that can show up during these tests; proving often for the first time in your life that these hated symptoms finally have a definite dietary connection.

Symptoms to look out for during testing can be anything from a recurrence of symptoms you are familiar with, to a bloated stomach, wind, headache, belching, or vague feelings of wooziness. If you get any of these, then put that food in the 'Under Suspicion' column and write beside it 'belching' or whatever symptom you experienced, along with the date, so that you will remember when to re-test. When you re-test that food five days later, and if the same belching or other symptom appears, put that food in the Forbidden Foods column.

You will continue testing in the above fashion until you identify all your food allergens.

Testing for allergens

Caution: If you are prone to asthma or epilepsy or have a severe psychiatric disorder, it is essential that any programme of testing, whether for tobacco or food allergy, should only be followed under strict medical supervision.

The multiple food test

Not for the faint-hearted, but it certainly can be a short cut. Instead of laboriously testing one food every 90 minutes, try a four or five-food test. Ideally these should be foods which are unlikely to prove allergenic (say, vegetables, but this is not always the case). You would eat the five portions at the one sitting, applying the same principles as before – taking the pulse before eating and then every 30 minutes thereafter until 90 minutes have passed.

If no symptoms or pulse change, then these four or five foods can be passed as 'Safe'. However, and this is where the frustration can set in, if it transpires that the combined foods do in fact affect your pulse, then you are almost back to square-one as you will have to re-test each of the foods individually at a later date (minimum 5 days later). So, although it can be a short cut if no reaction occurs – thereby clearing as 'Safe' several foods in one go – it can set you back a bit if the meal proves allergenic. It is perhaps a technique best left until you are well into the testing, when you have a large list of safe foods and any setback won't be too troublesome.

The add-one food tests

Another method of testing foods which makes it just that bit easier to tolerate is by testing proven 'Safe' foods at each meal with the simple addition of one new food.

Once you have cleared the foods as being safe, the addition of ONE other food to the 'safe' meal is a valid means of testing that additional food. If you are therefore safe with potatoes, beef, and gravy, you may have that meal with the new food (peas) and any positive pulse movements will mean you are allergic to the peas. This variation on single food testing can make the life of the food allergic many times more pleasant during this difficult testing period.

As you remove the offending items from your diet, your estimate of your lowest morning reading will change, until you arrive at your true minimal pulse reading. When this is reached you must remember that, as long as your diet is free from allergenic foods, and you do not have an illness, your 'at rest' pulse range during the day should not exceed 16 beats above your morning's reading. It is normal for the healthy pulse to increase during the day, but if it increases above 16 beats over your morning reading, you have been exposed to an allergen, whether food, drink, or inhalant.

Testing liquids

When testing liquids such as tea, coffee, milk, raw juices or even tap water, there is a quicker method which you can apply.

Again, take your pulse before the test. Then swirl the liquid around in your mouth, holding it under your tongue with your head slightly tilted back, and retaining it there for one full minute before swallowing.

You then only need to take your pulse (for the usual full minute's reading) at 15 minute intervals, three times. That is;

(i)   Take your pulse before the drink, then;
(ii)   15 minutes after drinking
(iii) 30 minutes after drinking
(iv)   45 minutes after drinking

You may consider that testing tap water is being somewhat over-cautious, but it is not uncommon for tap water to have small amounts of pesticides in it, as well as other adulterants such as lead, which can indeed influence the pulse.

You should remember that, as your testing progresses and your normal diet is split into safe and unsafe foods, so then will the need for testing reduce as you gather more and more information about the way your diet is affecting you as an individual. The most testing always takes place at the beginning and diminishes as you progress through the foods, until you are satisfied that you have covered all the foods you would normally be exposed to.

The Sublingual/pulse test

A direct challenge test: only the actual eating of a food can improve on this method and the testing is very much faster. But you must avoid all your allergenic foods and other substances for 5 days before testing.

You should either fast (nothing to eat, only distilled water to drink) for five days, commencing this testing on the 5th. Alternatively, you can eat a very restricted diet (intending to avoid all your allergenic foods) such as a single fruit for the entire period, or no more than two fruits. These can be selected from grapes, pears or apples.

Stick strictly to this limited regimen for the 5 days and commence testing on the 5th. Be aware that this sort of cleansing diet will undoubtedly incur withdrawal symptoms, so you should be alert to this.

Method: a drop of a liquid extract of the food or substance to be tested is placed sub-lingually (i.e.under the patient's tongue). This method allows for a swift delivery of the substance to the bloodstream.

You should be alert to pulse or symptom change and, if nothing has happened after 10 minutes, the food can be declared safe. Use the same pulse-taking method as before, watching for a change of 8 or more beats, either up or down, or watch out for any symptoms returning.

Some practitioners doubt the pulse technique's validity and state that there can be several false-positives (whereby a positive reaction may occur which later proves to be false) or false-negatives (whereby a negative reaction occurs but the substance proves later to be troublesome to the patient).

There can be reasons for these, however. A pulse rise with no obvious symptom response only means that the patient is UNAWARE of any physiological reaction, though one may still be taking place. Symptoms of food allergy such as a rise or drop in blood pressure may not be evident to the patient and therefore he might dismiss the food as being safe despite a change in pulse rate. Some practitioners consider that if the patient was not troubled by any symptom then the positive pulse reaction was a false-positive. The mere fact that the pulse was affected in the first place is evidence of a physiological reaction, and whether there are obvious symptoms alongside the pulse change does not matter; the pulse – the heart – has been affected, therefore the food must be viewed as 'unsafe' and the test positive.

If there is no pulse change, yet the patient feels something, these practitioners might classify the no-change pulse as being a false-negative. But the fact a reaction occurred at all was enough for the patient to identify the food as unsafe, therefore it did indeed achieve the desired result: positive identification of an allergen.

The only true test is the actual consuming of the substance and looking for definite symptoms. The sub-lingual method is the next best thing to eating the food.

The tobacco allergy test (sub-lingual)

You can test yourself for tobacco allergy by stopping smoking for five days and on the fifth day getting someone else to blow cigarette smoke into a cupful of water, until the water turns brown.

Put one drop of the liquid under your tongue and slightly tilt your head back. Hold it there for a full minute and a half. If you are allergic to tobacco smoke, you should within a few minutes get such a strong reaction that you will most certainly never wish to smoke again!

If you are prone to asthma or epilepsy or have a severe psychiatric disorder, it is essential that any programme of testing, whether for tobacco or food allergy, should only be followed under strict medical supervision.

17.

Case Histories

I thank Charlotte Gerson for allowing me to publish several case histories of people who have recovered their health using the Gerson Therapy. I present these cases together with some of my own.

Those patients who followed the Gerson diet did so for the 18 months to 2 year period normally required (a longer adherence to the diet is sometimes needed in very severe cases). The Gerson Therapy is a well-established method of recovery, based on Nature Cure principles. I present in the Recovery Programme later a diet that is very similar to the Gerson, as well as an explanation of the more intensive Gerson Therapy.

Among the following cases are some where mere identification of the problem foods has served to relieve the distress of the patient. Whilst such short-term relief is welcome, it should be recognised that mere avoidance is not the full answer for many people, and it would require the long term diet fully to recover from their 'food allergy' condition.

I would be doing a great disservice to the countless patients suffering from the food allergy condition if I were to wait the 4 or 5 years required to build up a catalogue of recovered patients who have achieved parasite/symptom eradication by diet and temperature control, before publishing. The number of patients with obvious food allergy symptoms who have recovered under the Gerson Therapy is in itself evidence that the Nature Cure approach works. I will produce a book of case histories in due course.

By publishing now I can help readers start immediately on the programme of recovery from their food allergy condition.

★ ★ ★

Mrs S.C. was a competitive swimmer. She complained of painful ears. Her doctor had prescribed drugs which did not help.

She was advised to alter her diet to have a fresh fruit breakfast, a salad at lunch, cooked vegetables in the evening, no meat but occasional fish.

She had to cut out tea and coffee. She reported that after two weeks she thought she had a brain tumour as the pain increased. After a further few weeks the pain began to subside and she hasn't had any pain in her ears since.

★ ★ ★

Marie H. was 56 years old. She had suffered for years with puffy, swollen eyes in the morning; she would sometimes have to wait until the afternoon for the swelling to go down before she could venture out. When she went to the toilet there was a lot of blood and mucus. It became so bad that she became very fearful. She was still holding down a part-time job but if she had to run to the toilet in an emergency, and it was occupied, she would often have an 'accident' which proved highly embarrassing. Her social life became non-existent and she was virtually afraid to go out.

She noticed that she was very stiff in the morning and had great difficulty bending her body to sit down. Her husband had to help her. She went to her doctor, who made a telephone call and arranged to admit her to hospital. She had a Barium meal and bowel X-rays. She was later diagnosed as having ulcerative colitis. She was given drugs but they didn't help and she developed pain all over her body and had great difficulty sleeping.

She was advised to cut out entirely all dairy products, of which she ate a lot. She had to eliminate all tinned and processed foods. She was advised to eat two raw salads per day. After about three weeks she started to feel better. Her sleeping improved greatly. She stuck rigidly to the Nature Cure diet and reported that the difference was 'unbelievable'.

Her symptoms disappeared and she could now sit and bend with ease. Her family remarked on how well she looked.

★ ★ ★

Dr. W. is a retired medical doctor who now lives in France. He suffered from severe asthma, sinusitis, rhinorrhea (nasal discharge), as well as being overweight. By avoiding foods to which he proved allergic and following a Nature Cure dietary regimen, he cleared all his symptoms entirely, as well as losing 2 stones in weight. Having witnessed the improvement made possible by dietary change alone, he qualified as a clinical ecologist and says that if he had his time over again he would undoubtedly choose diet as his first method of treatment.

★ ★ ★

Master J, aged 4 years, was hyperactive: he had non-stop energy. He was difficult to control, became violent at times and bedwetting was a problem. Constantly thirsty, he showed an allergy to cola, of which he drank a lot, as well as to sweets, chocolate and dairy products. After 3 weeks avoidance, there was a great change in his condition. His bedwetting, anxiety and violence disappeared. He became rational to speak to, where before he was irrational.

★ ★ ★

Miss L.B. was aged 75 and retired. She was shown to be allergic to dairy products, alcohol, house dust, pollen and grass (hayfever symptoms). Her symptoms of sneezing and tickly throat, watery eyes and nose stopped after two weeks avoidance and, as a bonus, she lost half a stone in three weeks.

★ ★ ★

Debra was 31, married with no children. She suffered from many allergies, which started when she was a hairdresser. She would itch all over.

She noticed that every time she went near chemicals such as bleach, her chest used to tighten and her eyes swell. The doctor diagnosed asthma and eczema and she was given an inhaler for the asthma and cream for the eczema. Her symptoms got worse as time went on. Her skin became very inflamed and she had difficulty sleeping because of the itching. When she did get to sleep it would only be for an hour or so because her chest would tighten and she would have to use her inhaler. Her diet was white bread, butter, burgers on toast, tinned foods, chocolate; in fact, she admitted, all the wrong things.

She was advised to throw away her creams and slowly decrease the use of the inhaler. She was told not to eat red meat, dairy products, white bread, white flour, pastry, sweets, chocolate, cakes, lemonade etc., – her usual fare. She had to stop drinking alcohol and was told to eat one large raw salad per day and as much fresh fruit as possible, as well as unsalted nuts.

Three weeks after starting the diet her skin became far worse, although her asthma didn't. She was told that this was just a 'healing crisis' and that she should persevere.

Daily there was slow improvement in her symptoms. After 6 to 8 weeks she showed great improvement. Her rash started to disappear, she lost about 10 lbs in weight. After 3-4 months all her symptoms had virtually gone and she had lost a stone and a half.

★ ★ ★

Mrs Doris C. suffered badly from sinusitis as well as rheumatic twinges. Her headaches would waken her in the early hours of the morning. Drugs eased the pain but made her stomach queasy, and she recognised that they did nothing to find the cause of her problem. She eliminated milk, sugar, alcohol and meat. An improvement started two and a half months later and continued slowly. Her headaches eventually disappeared entirely as did her rheumatic twinges. She says she still catches colds and 'flu, but with nowhere near the regularity she once did.

★ ★ ★

Marge Lemly suffered from heart disease and emphysema. In 1976 she had a nervous breakdown, and a heart attack with sharp chest pains, and was put on oxygen. She was unable to move and had extreme breathing difficulties. Her doctors prescribed digitalis, nitroglycerine and valium.

She was offered but refused, enderol. She lost 76 lbs in weight. She began the Gerson therapy in October 1979, regained weight and was alive and well at last contact twelve years later, in 1991.

★ ★ ★

Dr. James Clark had non-healing infections, arrhythmia (abnormal heart rate) and insomnia. In 1963 he suffered an ankle injury that would not heal. He had 13 operations and grafts which also would not heal.

After a year in hospital, his leg was removed below the knee. He continued to have infections, was given drugs and antiobiotics but still suffered arrhythmias, stomach distress, confusion, headaches and couldn't concentrate. He despaired of living and was admitted to a psychiatric hospital. He began the Gerson therapy in February 1978, recovered fully and today is alive and well.

★ ★ ★

Elizabeth Birdwell suffered poor health in early life, with many problems. Her mother had been prescribed drugs during pregnancy. Multiple Sclerosis was diagnosed in December 1973. Bartter's Syndrome was diagnosed. She also had confirmed hypothyroidism, hypoglycaemia, multiple allergies, early kidney failure, convulsions, profound exhaustion and muscle weakness.

She started the Gerson therapy in May 1984. There was steady improvement. She recovered fully to work as a model, attend University and get married. She was well at last contact in 1991, 7 years after starting the therapy.

★ ★ ★

Susan Adams had spreading melanoma (highly malignant tumour). She had moles removed from her right wrist. Malignant melanoma was confirmed by an outside hospital in January 1980. Three pathologists from the University of California agreed on the diagnosis. The tumour spread into right axilla (armpit) and was surgically cut out. The cancer continued spreading.

She began the Gerson therapy in November 1980 and achieved complete recovery. She had a recurrence after pregnancy, but recovered again.

★ ★ ★

Jacquie Davison (who recounted her full story in the book *Cancer Winner*) had tumours all over her head, neck, abdomen, diaphragm, arms and legs. Her abdomen bloated to 30lbs. Her doctor gave her no more than three weeks to live and she was advised her death would be swift and certain. She gave away most of her possessions and made her own funeral dress.

Her family encouraged her onto the Gerson therapy. She had many 'healing crises' but made a full recovery and is well 23 years later. Her book has just been reprinted.

★ ★ ★

Identical twins, Mary and Martha Ormesher, were diagnosed as having a fatal disease, Takayasu's Arteritis (Pulseless Disease). It started with Mary in 1978, when she was 16. She had an infection, diarrhoea, severe headaches, pain on breathing, extreme chest pains. Her doctor, Dr. Johnson, found no blood pressure or pulse in her right arm. Takayasu's was diagnosed. This diagnosis as confirmed by an outside clinic (the Mayo Clinic) in February 1979. She was given prednisone. Dr. Roland Johnson (Diplomate: American Board of Internal Medicine) said: 'This is a uniformly malignant and fatal arteritis.' A few months later, her twin sister Martha had the same symptoms and was similarly diagnosed.

Mary began the Gerson therapy in June 1980. Martha began in August. As well as the Gerson, they took some herbs. There was steady improvement. From a 'certain' death sentence, both girls fully recovered and are active, now 20 years later.

★ ★ ★

Melva Blackburn, 83 at the time of writing, had diabetes, arthritis, Alzheimer's Disease, kidney and adrenal disease, Cushing's Syndrome, etc. She had medical problems from 1944 onwards and was treated till 1979. She was given drugs for her heart (coronary artery) disease, drugs to treat diabetes (from 1965). She had poor control of her legs and feet, Cushing's Syndrome (adrenal disease, obesity, fatigue, weakness, osteoporosis, oedema, infections), pneumonia twice a year, an enlarged liver, arthritis in all joints, anxiety, ataxia (unsteady gait), confusion, aphasia (speech difficulty), Alzheimer's was diagnosed. She had been on drugs for many years and had many operations for her problems.

She began the Gerson therapy in October 1979 and rapidly improved. All diseases went without drugs. She astounded her doctors and remains active and well 21 years later.

★ ★ ★

Marilyn Dent had 11 operations in 11 years. She suffered from migraines, tachycardia, hypoglycaemia and mental illness. She had a hysterectomy and various exploratory operations. Surgery injured the sciatic nerve giving her constant severe pain and sharp intermittent pain from head to feet. She was given many drugs for her various symptoms, suffered a nervous breakdown and was admitted to a psychiatric ward.

She began the Gerson therapy in October 1977 and showed rapid improvement. She came off all drugs and, at last contact in 1991, was in good condition and living a normal life.

★ ★ ★

David Nelson (son of Bill Nelson, below) was diagnosed as having 'hopeless' astrocytoma brain cancer in January 1986. He had a grand mal seizure. Surgery removed 50% of the tumour, which was described as lemon-sized with many 'crabgrass roots' into the brain remaining. A biopsy confirmed astrocytoma (brain tumour), and doctors gave him between 2 and 12 months to live. He began the Gerson therapy in April 1986. Four MRI scans in 3 years showed reduction and then disappearance of the tumour. He was alive and well 12 years later despite being careless in working with chemicals, which produced a recurrence. He is now recovering.

★ ★ ★

Bill Nelson, father of David Nelson, suffered from Candida (yeast infection) and was prone to chemical sensitivity. After a restaurant meal in 1977 he had a hard time breathing. He was given drugs without any diagnosis. In 1978, he had the first of five sinus operations. These didn't help. He couldn't breathe and was given more drugs, including antibiotics. He had white fungus spots on the mouth and private parts and probably had yeast infection in the lungs. 60mg cortisone daily gave no relief. He couldn't sleep. He was on continuous oxygen. He began Gerson in April 1986, with immediate improvement. Completely recovered, he built a house and remains well 12 years later.

★ ★ ★

Lara Bradley had breast cancer biopsied in 1984, with nodules on breast and liver, plus medically diagnosed herpes simplex, Epstein-Barr, hypoglycaemia, chronic fatigue syndrome, histo-plasmosis (virus from birds) and severe depression. She began Gerson therapy May 1984. Fully recovered, she is well 14 years later. She has written a book under the pen-name Alexandra Lennox, which is to be published soon.

* * *

Bill Goerdes, who passed away recently aged nearly 100, was diagnosed with severe rheumatoid arthritis and bleeding stomach ulcers in 1941. New York Presbyterian Medical Center X-rays showed his spine fused top to bottom with rheumatoid arthritis. He was offered no hope. Beginning Gerson therapy with Dr. Gerson in October 1941, his ulcers were gone in six weeks. He was able to return to light work in seven and a half months and commenced heavier duties in 14 months.

Completely restored to health by the therapy he was well and active for almost 60 years. It is interesting to note that Charlotte Gerson confirmed to me that Bill, whose spine was 'fused top to bottom' had his 'bones restored and separated'!

* * *

Deanna Powell had severe rheumatoid arthritis and was bedridden in 1976. She suffered constant pain and stiffness. All her joints were swollen; her elbows, knees and most fingers bent and frozen. She had bony deformities and walked with great difficulty. She had heart palpitations, laboured breathing and was pale, anaemic and had hypoglycaemia. She was taking 15-20 aspirins daily but still had pain and insomnia. She began Gerson in May 1978. In six weeks the pain was gone and most lumps had started to dissolve. All problems were resolved except a few joints which were not quite clear. She got married and had a family, experiencing a recurrence of her symptoms after pregnancy, from which she recovered. She took up water skiing and is well 20 years later.

18.

Eating Naturally Can Cure

A lady from England telephoned me in 1995, looking for the number of a Nature Cure Clinic – the Kingston Clinic – that was once situated near to where I live in Edinburgh.

Advising her that it had recently closed, I asked her why she was looking for it. She replied: 'My mother went there in 1946 when she was told by her doctor that she would have to have a kidney removed. She was put on a diet at the Kingston Clinic. She died recently, aged 86 and with both her kidneys intact. I am having heart trouble and I want to follow the same kind of advice as my mother got.'

These word-of-mouth reports are common among people familiar with natural healing. However, if you were to relate them to your doctor, he would dismiss them as being merely 'anecdotal'.

How can such an event be anything other than 'anecdotal' when one doesn't travel around on a daily basis with clinicians, X-rays, ultra-sound equipment etc., logging each and every step of the way? The patient is urgently seeking proper advice, and if he or she gets it at a Nature Cure clinic, or achieves recovery by adhering to a completely natural diet, then that is a success. To dismiss it as 'anecdotal' is a piece of nonsense, prompted by a mixture of embarrassment at being unable to achieve the healing, and indignation.

However had that 'anecdote' which the lady passed to me, been heard from the lips of a doctor, it would surely have taken on the mantle of a 'case study' and have become very valid indeed...

Doctors are quick to dismiss recoveries by diet as having 'no evidence'. Yet these same doctors embrace and recommend psychiatry. Somehow it has become part of medical training whilst, unbelievably, there is no evidence that it works, certainly not evidence that meets the stringent requirements of proof that they demand of nutritional medicine.

I relate elsewhere the story from *Nutrition and Your Mind* by Dr. George Watson of a lady who had spent years on the psychiatrist's couch, and thousands upon thousands of dollars, in an unsuccessful effort to cure her depression.

Yet when she was tested for food allergies and these culprit foods removed, her depression lifted 'as if by magic'!

The evidence that Nature can heal is overwhelming. It happens in the wild without ceremony. It happens to you and me on a regular basis, our little cuts healing without significant attention being given. There are many examples in man of serious health disorders being remedied by applying natural methods, but widespread knowledge of these is not encouraged by the medical profession, which will regularly dismiss such events as either gross exaggeration of the true facts or as hokus pokus.

Whilst Nature Cure clinics are to be found in many countries, the best documented 'evidence' of all must lie in the camp of the Gerson therapy. Not only do they achieve wonderful results in healing, but they do it in such a way as never to be accused of 'fiddling' their records.

There have been several attempts to discredit the Gerson therapy, mostly by those who would lose financially if it were to be universally accepted. But to discredit the Gerson therapy, you would have to be able to discredit Nature Cure, and to do that you would have to discredit Nature: a very difficult task indeed.

To ensure they couldn't be accused of interfering with their records, Gerson therapists insist that all patients are given expert diagnoses by outside orthodox medical hospitals before they are taken onto the programme. With an 'orthodox' medical diagnosis to start with, no-one can later accuse them of inventing the original condition. No-one can say, once a cancer has been cured, that it couldn't have been cancer in the first place, if outside diagnosis exists from the start.

Their dietary programme is very intensive. It should be followed for anything from 18 months to two or three years and even beyond in difficult cases. They have their own clinic and hospital but many people around the world have succeeded in applying the dietary approach in their own homes without the need to travel to their hospital facilities in Mexico.

The records of full recovery from terminal illnesses held on file at the Gerson clinic are very convincing and would stand up to close scrutiny by any medical investigator.

Orthodox medicine in the U.S.A. – the American Medical Association – labelled Dr. Max Gerson under the 'Frauds and Fables' category, despite overwhelming evidence to show that his programme of diet treatment worked. One can only assume there would be loss of face as well as financial support by the drug companies if mere diet and not drugs could achieve such fascinating results.

An indicator of how orthodox medicine can view Nature Cure treatments comes in the form of a story that naturopath Keki Sidhwa told me in 1995, when I undertook a 30-day fast under his supervision at his Shalimar clinic in Frinton, England.

When he was training in naturopathy at the Kingston Clinic (the same clinic mentioned earlier), Keki shared a flat with an orthodox medical student. They lived in separate rooms. They got on very well and, interested, the medical student would often ask Keki just what natural healing involved and how it worked. Keki, naturally, was happy to let the medical student know just what he was taught in his training. They often chatted to each other about their respective studies.

However, suddenly and without warning, Keki returned from his studies one day to find a note had been pushed under his door. It was from the medical student and it had words on it to the effect that he didn't want to speak to Keki ever again!

Keki was stunned. They had not crossed swords. They had not fallen out. Keki could not understand why the medical student should act in this way. Every attempt by Keki to find out what the matter was, failed. The medical student soon left his accommodation and Keki was not to find out the reason.

Several years later, Keki was in the street when he heard someone shout out his name. It was the former medical student. He ran over to Keki and apologised for what had happened. He told Keki that he had now qualified as a doctor. Keki congratulated him. The medical student explained that his family in India had saved up a fortune to send him to Britain to train as a doctor and all his family were putting their faith in him qualifying. He couldn't let them down – it would have destroyed his family.

He explained that the reason he had to stop seeing Keki was because everything Keki was saying was making so much sense that the medical student was beginning to question his own medical training. He feared he might abandon his entire medical career if he listened to Keki any longer!

Whilst Keki's original training was Nature Cure and therefore diet-oriented, he took a great interest in fasting as a means of assisting Nature achieve her healing. Animals in the wild instinctively fast when they are ill, and they recover. Man, on the other hand, is prompted by his doctor and family, to 'eat to keep up strength'. Eating when ill, when the body doesn't demand food, impedes recovery rather than assists it. There have been innumerable cases of therapeutic fasting helping extremely ill patients recover, (I plan to cover that in a future book).

Let us look now at what 'merely' changing your diet can do for you and your health.

The Gerson therapy

The story of the Gerson therapy is a wonderful, inspiring one, and at the same time extremely sad, because of the way its discoverer was treated by the medical profession in America.

Max Gerson M.D., was born in Germany in 1881. A migraine sufferer, he was told by his doctor that he would have to live with it. Undeterred, Gerson, after reading of an Italian doctor who had successfully controlled his migraine by diet, experimented with his own and found that, by eliminating some foods and eating raw fruits and vegetables, his migraine disappeared.

He later applied the same dietary principles that he had learned, with great success, to his own migraine patients. One day, one of his migraine sufferers reported to Dr. Gerson that his lupus vulgaris – or skin T.B. – was going away. Dr. Gerson expressed disbelief, because everyone knew that lupus was an 'incurable' disease. But the evidence was there before his very eyes – the lupus was indeed healing. He reasoned, rightly it turned out, that the body, on this natural-food diet, was healing itself. Other lupus patients soon came to see him. They too were cured. Gerson found that patients with secondary ailments such as arthritis and other so-called incurable illnesses, had these afflictions similarly helped by the diet.

His treatment soon reached the ears of a Professor Sauerbruch in Austria, a world-famous thoracic surgeon and tuberculosis authority. He showed great interest in Gerson's claims to cure lupus and invited a trial with lupus patients at his Austrian clinic.

After a few weeks, Sauerbruch, with a heavy heart, sat down to write a telegram to Gerson to tell him that the diet had failed; it was not a success after all. Hugely disappointed, Sauerbruch was on his way back through his clinic after sending the telegram when he noticed a nurse climbing the stairs to the part of the building which housed the lupus patients.

She was carrying a tray with beer, sausages and other forbidden items.

Sauerbruch immediately called her to stop and demanded to know what she was doing. 'I am taking these poor lupus patients something nice to eat, I feel so sorry for them.' In a rage, Sauerbruch smashed the tray to the floor and vowed to tighten up the strict dietary rules he was insisting on. He immediately sat down and penned another telegram apologising for the earlier one and advising him he was starting again.

Sauerbruch's clinical trial of Gerson's dietary treatment proved an astonishing success, with lasting cures in 446 out of 450 lupus sufferers! This event is related in Sauerbruch's own autobiography, *Master Surgeon*.

Instead of being awarded the Nobel Prize as might have been expected,

Gerson was called before a court, by irritated and doubtless embarrassed physicians, to defend his treatment. He won the case, but this resistance by orthodox medicine against a successful dietary treatment was to prove an on-going feature for the rest of his life.

When he fled to America to avoid Hitler's hounding of the Jews, his diet had now become successful in curing very many terminally ill cancer patients. He had the biopsies performed by outside hospitals to ensure the patients' original diagnoses of cancer could not later be brought into doubt. X-rays taken before and after treatment, showing tumours gone, were available to all visiting physicians. He was so keen to share his success that he invited the American Medical Association down to his clinic.

They came and saw all his records, and left without saying much. Despite all Gerson's marvellous success stories with extremely difficult cases who had been sent home to die and had now fully recovered under his treatment, the AMA labelled him under the 'Frauds and Fables' category!

The AMA, I have read elsewhere, receive massive funding from the huge pharmaceutical companies in the form of advertising revenue: millions upon millions of dollars per year. Perhaps it was considered that, as Gerson used no drugs whatsoever, if the treatment took off, it would threaten the drug industry and consequently the AMA itself. That is an extremely valid and on-going indictment of these wealthy drug companies. Clearly, if Nature Cure took the place of drug taking, the companies would virtually be wiped out, as would the massive funds paid each year to the AMA.

It was made a crime in California to treat cancer by diet, and Gerson had to open a clinic over the border in Mexico to avoid being taken to court.

That did not stop many medical students wanting to study under him, but they were told in not too many words, that if they did so their futures would be in jeopardy. Other doctors, aware of Gerson's success, would be jeopardising their licence to practise if they treated their own cancer patients with the diet. They would only instruct very close patients, whom they could trust to keep quiet, in the diet. Many an American medical doctor has cured himself of cancer by following the diet, despite not being allowed to give such benefit to the patients in his care.

The remarkable achievements of the diet in completely turning around often 'terminal' cancers are in themselves outstanding, but the manner in which the cancers can be healed is even more fascinating.

Beata Bishop recalls in *A Time to Heal* that, after she had been on the therapy for approximately 18 months, she realised that there was a lump in her groin which, naturally, greatly worried her. It was decided to operate to remove the lump and have a pathologist report on it.

To her great surprise, it turned out that the tumour had indeed been isolated, out of harm's way within the body. The live tumour had shrunk and was enclosed in a fifteen millimetre thick capsule! The healing power, in its incredible wisdom had not only arrested the further spread of the disease, but had 'cornered' the very nucleus of the tumour and walled it off so that it might do no more harm! To quote Beata on discovering the thickness of the encapsulation of the tumour: 'Fifteen? That's almost bullet-proof!'.

The lump was then surgically removed, purely as a precaution.

The lump told its own story: it was evident that the cancer was to all intents and purposes, 'outwith' the body. It had been encased in a calcified cocoon. It had been defeated, and well and truly trapped.

However, what would have happened if she had not had it surgically removed and it had remained in her body? Because the live cancerous cells in the very heart of the encapsulation were also surrounded by dead cells, one can hypothesise that these live cells were on borrowed time and would eventually have met with the same fate as the dead cells surrounding them and that slowly they too would have died off.

And the likely scenario after that would have been for the entire lump to have slowly dissolved and been removed from the body by the body's own eliminatory capabilities, as in *The Grape Cure,* a book written by Basil Shackleton. Shackleton related that, after six weeks on nothing but grapes and water, his tumour was dissolved by the healing power of the fruit and carried out of his body in his urine: He had the excreted mass confirmed by a London pathologist as being the dissolved tumour.

The above happened to Beata because her healing power – which is no different from yours or mine – had been supplied with the correct nutrition so that it could work at its greatest efficiency. It obviously had not been working efficiently in the first place, or she would not have developed the cancer.

A feature writer for the *New York Enquirer* heard about Gerson and his 'cancer diet' and set out to prove him a fraud. Robert Lichello (it was he who suggested the change of name to the *National Enquirer*) considered that Gerson must have been fleecing his vulnerable cancer patients and making a fortune. He started his own investigation.

Instead of finding a con man charging a fortune for some elixir that didn't work, Lichello found a quiet, dedicated doctor, often treating patients free of charge, or charging very little, and getting remarkable results. It wasn't long before Lichello, instead of branding him a fraud as did the AMA, started championing him, and even wrote a book about Gerson and his genuine cancer cures. He wrote *Cancer? Think Curable; The Gerson Therapy,* under the pen name S.J. Haught.

The Gerson regimen is a highly-intensive natural approach whereby the patient drinks 13 half-pint glasses of freshly pressed raw organic vegetable and fruit juices each day, as well as an abundance of other fruits and vegetables and a special soup.

A dietary treatment for cancer similar to the Gerson therapy is, surprisingly enough, widely recognised by the Dutch government and is widely available in hospitals throughout Holland. The Moerman Diet was 'invented' by a Dutch G.P. called Cornelis Moerman, who, in the 1930s – after Gerson discovered his dietary treatment – arrived at his own dietary treatment for cancer. His and Gerson's diets are very similar, but in my opinion Gerson's has the edge by virtue of the fact they have extensive documentation of patients that recovered.

In a book by Ruth Jochems, *The Moerman Cancer Diet*, the actual process of encapsulating a tumour is dealt with as something well established, rather than out of the ordinary. To quote:

Dr. Moerman's natural cure divides the healing process into three stages:

1. Stopping the growth of the tumour.
2. Walling off the tumour by encapsulation.
3. Breaking the tumour down.

To make the method work the patient needs three things:

1. The diet.
2. The vitamin supplements
3. A will of iron.

If you've got all three, you can cure yourself!

So the fascinating encapsulation of a tumour, which would probably make the eyes of an 'ordinary' cancer doctor stand out on stalks, is a well-recognised phenomenon in Nature Cure and seems to be expected, no matter where the dietary therapy is applied.

The process is invariable because the elements that are involved – man, natural foods and Nature – are the same, no matter where in the world you may be.

The research in this book showing that an intensive natural diet can raise body temperature adds a new dimension to the explanation of how these diets can achieve such wonderful recoveries from ill health.

Pottenger's cats

Frances M. Pottenger, M.D. was an American doctor who made significant contributions to the role nutrition plays in maintaining good health and, indeed, in correcting ill health.

His classic ten-year study of 900 cats gave a priceless insight into the consequences of poor nutrition upon health and, probably more importantly, on the effect of nutrition on the health of the offspring of the cats.

He fed one group of cats on pasteurised (heated) milk, cooked meat and cod liver oil. These animals developed allergies, were generally in poor health, and had skeletal deformities, as well as exhibiting homosexual tendencies.

Further, each successive generation became poorer in health, producing smaller and weaker litters with low birth weight animals.

He fed another group of cats with the same food, but this time the meat was raw and the milk UNpasteurised (raw). These animals were healthy, had good skeletal structure and were normal and happy in their behaviour. There was no homosexuality and their offspring too were healthy through successive generations, unlike the cooked-food group which showed all manner of disease symptoms.[121] Pottenger states:

> In giving cats cooked meat and milk, they develop all kinds of allergies. They sneeze, wheeze and scratch. They are irritable, nervous and do not purr. First deficient generation allergic cats produce second generation kittens with greater incidence of allergies, and by the third generation, the incidence is almost 100 percent.[122]

I believe that the scratching, the wheezing, and the allergies could be due to migratory parasites interfering with normal function in the skin, lungs, and anywhere else in the body. The cooked, unnatural diet the animals were fed would undoubtedly have lowered their body temperature and their state of health, and made them easy prey for parasites.

The Hunza people

Perhaps the most famous example of excellence in the health of man must be the Hunza people, properly referred to as the Hunzakuts, who live in a remote part of the Himalayas. When Sir Robert McCarrison, an eminent English surgeon visited this remote tribespeople in the 1920s, he came back full of stories of the fabulous health and physiques that were constant throughout their community. Where they lived was so cut off from the outside that they had to be self-sufficient in all that they did – and ate.

McCarrison had never seen a people who were so completely free of all disease and ill health. They lived very long and active lives. Men fathered children in their 90s and anyone of 80 was considered merely middle-aged!

After extensive research and experiment, McCarrison was able to prove conclusively that their supreme health, vitality and freedom from disease were no mere flukes, but were totally due to their natural diet. Furthermore, by feeding diseased rats the Hunza diet, their health was restored; further proof, if proof be needed, that the number one factor in health is, and always will be, diet.

McCarrison fed the Hunza diet to mice that he kept for such experimentation and found that these mice grew completely normally and had superb health. When he fed other mice the diets of various regions of India, where health problems were common, he was able to reproduce the health problems of those regions. Mice fed on a typical Calcutta diet developed the problems common in that city. A Madras-type diet and a Bombay diet produced the respective health defects of those places.

When McCarrison applied the appalling 'English' diet of tea, white toast and tinned foods, the mice thus fed developed poor fur, had little energy, fought with each other and were short lived: all indications that they were living a miserable existence. The mice fed on the Hunza diet became well-grown, with sleek shiny fur, strong and playful with each other, and long lived.

The supremely healthy Hunza diet[123] consisted of leafy green vegetables, fruits – chiefly apricots and mulberries – fresh and sun-dried, wholegrains, potatoes and other root vegetables; peas and beans, gram of chick pea, and other pulses, fresh, raw milk and buttermilk, or lassi, and meat only on very rare occasions. They drank water from the mountain glaciers.

It is a sad reflection on what might be considered 'progress' that the Hunza people – now accessible to outsiders and indulging in their visitors' foods – are starting to show signs of ill health that mirror our own industrialised nations' horrific catalogue of modern diseases.

To underline this recognised deterioration in so-called 'primitive' man's health after their being introduced to our 'modern' diet, I quote from *Nutrition and Physical Degeneration* by Weston A. Price D.D.S., who travelled the globe comparing the health of primitive civilisations:

If any one impression of our experiences were to be selected as particularly vivid, it would be the contrast between the health and ruggedness of the primitives in general and that of the foreigners who have entered their country. That their superior ruggedness was not racial became evident when, through contact with modern civilisation, degenerative processes developed.

19.

We Can Heal Our Selves

The power to heal our bodies is within all of us. We are brought up to revere doctors and instinctively seek them when our health is in trouble. But have you considered just how far a doctor's knowledge extends when it comes to *healing* illness?

Take an illness, arthritis for example, or depression, or acne, or fibrositis. Anyone attending their doctor with any of these, or a hundred plus similar disorders, will, in all likelihood, be given drugs, which will have only a temporary effect. The effect may be welcome relief, but when the drug wears off, the condition will still be there. In other words, the doctor will not have *cured* the condition. He will merely have administered temporary relief.

He or she will then administer that temporary relief over and over again, perhaps for many years, until the problem either clears up on its own, or until you die. The doctor will not have found the *cause* of, or indeed the *cure* for, any of these hundred diseases.

I am not alone in believing that the future of the world's health lies in nutritional medicine, not in the dispensing of drugs. The medical profession might be able to 'cure' a diseased kidney, by removing it from the body, but is that a true cure? I think not. They may be able to 'cure' cancer of the breast by slicing the breast from the woman's chest. But is that 'curing' the cancer?

Doctors give little attention to the cause of illnesses but concentrate all their efforts on finding an appropriate pharmaceutical product which will only go some way to providing temporary relief.

The logic in taking someone who has a health problem and, without finding and removing the cause, *adding* to that person's already-compromised system, toxic pharmaceutical products often over many years, simply is *not* good science!

This state of affairs, prevalent in most countries, is especially worrying because drugs are *not* tested on humans over the long-term (months and years), contrary to popular belief. We become long-term guinea pigs when the drug is passed as 'safe' and approved for sale to the public.

Eminent scientists and doctors around the world, including the late Linus Pauling – the only double Nobel Prize Winner – have become disillusioned with drugs and their toxic consequences.

The wonderful healing ability that we all have is given little leeway to perform its undoubted miracles in our modern society. We rely on the doctor or hospital to put right our many illnesses when more often than not, if the condition is left to run its course, it will heal of its own accord.

The body, having sustained and dealt with the 'attack' will be all the stronger for it. Think, for example, the 'immunity' one dose of an infection such as measles can confer on a patient, if the condition is allowed to run its course unimpeded by drugs.

The interference in Nature's attempts to recover health by the application of drugs is a backward step. Nature knows what it is doing in the healing department if only given the chance.

The true extent of Nature's healing powers is there for all to see – if we only look. The small cut, the tiny graze, they all heal and we don't even pay attention to them. But bigger, more ominous diseases can also be turned around from a seemingly terminal prognosis to total health. Often conditions that doctors will dismiss as being 'inoperable' or 'terminal' can be removed and health restored to the patient.

If you consider that referring to 'Nature Cure' sounds dated and smacks of Austrian health clinics of fifty or one hundred years ago, you have to realise you cannot get much more old fashioned than Nature – nor more powerful. Rip yourself away from the modern way of thinking, that every ill has a pill, and peer into the wonderful healing powers Nature is – or can be – capable of.

Let us look at an example of Nature performing her unseen, but absolutely beautifully-orchestrated miracle of healing. Let us see how a broken leg repairs itself. The following is from *How Nature Heals*:

If the bone of a man or any animal be broken, and the parts replaced, the presiding and guiding force of the animal economy – call it Nature or what you will – at once deposits a liquid substance over the entire surface of the bone, a short distance in opposite directions from the fracture. This liquid soon hardens into a bone-like substance and becomes a ring firmly attached to each section of the broken bone, and for a time affords the chief support whereby the damaged limb can be used. In due time the ends of the bone – which, perhaps, had been entirely severed – become united.

Nature establishes a circulation through its parts, whereby each part is again nourished; and the limb, having its broken bone reunited, is able to support the weight of the body without calling upon the strength of the bone ring which had been temporarily built around the fractured bone.

What happens? Nature, finding no doubt that all needless supports are a damage, proceeds to soften and absorb this bone ring until it is all removed except a slight portion for an eighth or a quarter of an inch about the point of fracture.

A similar and more familiar phenomenon is seen whenever and wherever the skin is broken; at once there is an exudation of blood; this coagulates upon exposure to the air, and forms an excellent airtight protection (a scab) to the injured part, which remains for a longer or shorter period, as may be needed, and when Nature has formed a new skin underneath, and the scab is no longer required, Nature proceeds to undermine and separate it; and while as long as it was needed it was firmly attached, so soon as no longer required, it falls off of its own weight.

Similarly, a sliver becomes imbedded in the flesh – a frequent accident. If a surgeon is at hand and removes it, well and good – Nature soon repairs the damage. If a surgeon is not at hand and the sliver is thus permitted to remain, Nature at once sets about a bit of fascinating engineering. First there is pain and inflammation; then follows a formation of pus; this in due time breaks down the tissues immediately surrounding the sliver, especially toward the surface of the limb. The pus increases, breaks through, runs out, and sooner or later carries the sliver with it. No surgeon needed![124]

You need only look at animals in the wild to witness Nature working unimpeded, when she is not being hampered in her efforts by medications or highly poisonous chemical drugs. The knitting of bones in wild animals occurs all the time, without splints or nurses or doctors. It is easy to understand how man can, with medical assistance from a hospital outpatient department, recover fully from a broken leg. It is less easy to grasp how such healing can be achieved in a dumb animal in the forest or jungle, without such help.

In his book *The Sex Life of Wild Animals* Eugene Burns provides us with the following brief account of the healing of broken bones in the wild.

One study on mammalian bone healing in the wild is truly amazing. Of ninety five opossum skeletons taken at random near Lawrence, Kansas, thirty nine had broken bones which had healed perfectly. Many had survived broken ribs and shoulders, some of these sustained, presumably, in competitive male fighting. One opossum had recovered from a total of two broken shoulders, eleven broken ribs (two of which had been broken twice) and a badly damaged vertebral column. Certainly, many of these injuries sustained by the opossum might have finished off heavier creatures. The recuperative power of a wild creature is enormous; broken legs slough off their decayed flesh and grow whole again, parasite-riddled organs heal, old-rotted tissues renew fresh and clean.

That destroys the usual argument that if you don't put a broken limb into a splint, it will heal awkwardly, imprecisely, or unevenly. Eugene Burns states that the broken bones healed perfectly. We are so used to doctors tending our wounds that we defend our own methods of repair against what might seem primitive. But primitive is Nature, and nothing matches Nature in her ability to heal.

Examples of such repairs have been collected from every animal species in wild nature. The animals' wounds heal and their broken bones knit without the 'advantage' of a surgeon or physician to set their broken bones or give them an anti-tetanus injection. They do not receive an anti-rabies vaccine, their wounds are not dressed or treated with antiseptics and no one gives them antibiotics.

Healing is a continuous process in Nature. She strives continually to attain full health. However, our daily artificial diets impede seriously the ability of the body to achieve full healing under every circumstance. We are healed all the time of minor injuries, to which we give no conscious attention. The many little scratches, cuts, bruises, twists and tears which we receive almost daily, but which are so insignificant that we do nothing about them, are quickly healed.

Sometimes the process is so rapid that a small injury of this kind is completely healed overnight. We mash a finger with a hammer, the tissues are bruised and mangled. In a day or two the finger is healed and the incident is forgotten although we have applied no supposed treatment. The healing of more serious injuries is accomplished with the same powers and processes by which these minor injuries are healed, the chief difference being that it takes more time.

Whilst animals in the wild, as stated by Eugene Burns, have recuperative powers that are 'enormous', you have to recognise that animals in the wild do not eat their foods out of packets and tins. They don't eat highly cooked and processed foods that have been chemically sprayed, and adulterated in order to prolong their shelf lives. Their diet is as Nature intended them to eat – natural and uncooked. They don't take toxic chemicals in the form of drugs as part of their diet whenever they fall ill, or continue to take them for months or years on end.

Man's recuperative powers also could be 'enormous' if he were to follow the example of animals and allow Nature to cure and not further burden his already-ill body with impediments to recovery such as drugs.

Drugs give the appearance of healing because they appear to remove a headache or other pain, if such symptoms appear occasionally. But if the pain reappears, the drugs become less and less capable of handling the problem, until eventually they do no good at all. Yet the doctor, aware that they worked once, often will prescribe drugs for months, even years on end. All the time residues of these drugs can accumulate in the body and cause unnoticed harm. All drugs are not automatically dispelled from the body as you might be advised.

A drug may 'remove' a headache; it does not remove the cause. The chances are that if you maintain the cause of that headache, whether it be bad diet, smoking, or alcohol, the headache will return. Your aim is to remove the cause and that is where nutritional medicine and naturopathy (natural healing) excel because we look at the patient's diet and lifestyle and adjust them accordingly. We seek to embrace the power of Nature's healing abilities; we seek to harness this massive power, not impede it.

Doctors are unaccustomed to watching Nature heal everyday occurrences; they consider that drugs can outwit Nature. Outwit? No. Interfere with? Certainly.

Most drugs have a short, temporary effect on symptoms, and then it wears off. The patient eventually needs to take more and more of the drug to experience the effect it originally had. Eventually however, the effectiveness the drug once displayed disappears and the taking of the medication simply becomes a habit. Despite the drug's effects waning dramatically, it will still be prescribed, often for years. What such long-term, daily poisoning does to the organism is anybody's guess, but the arrival of new symptoms as a result of this heavy load of medication is a common feature of such treatment. For these new symptoms, further drugs will be prescribed and so this farcical circumstance will go on - the familiar 'repeat prescription' scenario.

I remember only too well as a boy visiting my great-uncle, who was over 70, each night after his wife had died. As he now lived alone and had many symptoms of ill health to contend with, I had to ensure he was safe and didn't require anything. The number of pill bottles he had to sift through each night in order to complete his drug-taking, was, even to a boy, mind boggling! Despite the mass of drugs which his doctor instructed him to take, his symptoms were still with him. These drugs did not restore health at all. Indeed it breaks my heart to know what I could have done for him, knowing what I now know. The number of such people throughout the world who are in similar circumstances doesn't bear thinking about.

Many recoveries from ill health have been accomplished by the simple expedient of removing all drugs from the patient's bedside.

However, I should warn the reader that you should NOT suddenly stop taking any drugs that you are taking, without the full co-operation of your doctor. Such action, under certain circumstances, can be dangerous.

20.

Drugs Can Not Heal

We are all virtually programmed into calling on the doctor whenever we become ill. This conditioning is so well established that it is almost innate. There can indeed be merit in doing so, if for no other reason than to eliminate the possibility of serious disease and so achieve peace of mind.

The vast majority of 'illnesses' are quite minor and will clear up without the need for drugs. However, the 'I need some pill for my ailment' plea to the family doctor is almost automatic in our thinking.

The doctor might put iodine on a cut and cover it with a sticking plaster, but it is not the sticking plaster, or the iodine, or the doctor, who carries out the healing: the body repairs itself, healing from the inside, out, so that the cut closes completely.

All doctors accept that healing comes from within our own bodies. We all take the sight of a cut healing for granted, as we do the act of breathing. The ability to heal oneself is there within you, although some people heal faster than others. The reason for that centres around the health – the nutritional status – of the individual. Indeed, not only is healing reliant on a rich supply of nutrients to the entire system, but even within one person, different areas of the body can exhibit faster healing than others. That anomaly may be explained by the fact that the blood, carrying the healing nutrients, may have freer access to some areas than others.

If you are a slow healer, or if you have a chronic disease that has never fully healed, then you should seek to improve your nutrition in order to achieve recovery.

Although the body of a slow healer may well still be able to perform minor acts of healing, like a small cut or graze, more intensive healing for, say, a leg ulcer might take considerably longer – even years in some cases. If you indulge in an artificial (processed food) diet which makes life difficult for your own body's eliminatory functions, then you will expend extra energy in dealing with these incoming unnatural foodstuffs, energy that could be better used elsewhere, in healing for example.

If you have a lifetime of poor diet behind you, poor that is in natural fruits and vegetables, then your body's healing abilities will have been chronically compromised. This will account for the body's ability to do minor repairs, yet struggle to achieve healing in more serious conditions.

If one can restore one's health to that of a healthy person, then your ability to heal will also be that of a healthy person, and that can be done through vastly improving your diet over a sustained period of time.

Drugs may give the illusion of healing, but they do not heal. The majority of illnesses do not require drug intervention. Drugs may paralyse the site of the symptom and give freedom from pain whilst the body itself carries out the repair; or they may remove altogether – temporarily – the symptom, only for it to return in an even worse form when the drug wears off. This merry-go-round of drug taking to 'treat' a condition is the 'repeat prescription' syndrome with which most of us are only too familiar.

You will never remove the cause of a chronic condition by taking drugs. Temporary alleviation of the symptoms may be enough for many people. However, as there is overwhelming evidence that most modern diseases are diet-related, i.e. caused by poor diet, then unless you change your diet, you cannot hope to remove the true cause of your affliction.

Adding a toxic chemical – a drug – to your compromised body, whilst still indulging in the poor diet, cannot possibly remove the true cause of the condition. Instead of just having the sustained poor diet to contend with, your body now has unnatural toxic chemical compounds on top. As these drugs are often taken for weeks, months, or even decades on end, the toxic insult to your body adds even further to your miseries, and more and more health complications can arise. What happens when they do? You know the answer: more and more drugs.

We are unaccustomed to allowing our illnesses to run their own paths to recovery. Doctors themselves are unfamiliar with the process of letting the patient's disease run its own natural course. They are trained to administer drugs, but this perpetual drug prescribing interferes with the body's own healing powers. If a condition heals (and I do mean healing, not temporary suppression of the symptoms) whilst on drugs, it heals as a result of the body's own healing powers fighting through the effect of the drug. Except in true emergencies, where nature does not have the time to achieve repair, She should be allowed a chance to remedy the affliction.

Although the idea of refusing medicines at a time when a child is ill would put the fear of death into many parents, the truth of the matter is that the vast majority of conditions will recover of their own accord if Nature is allowed to take control.

Our medical practitioners are simply not taught to use Nature as their ally but instead pander to the patients' request for immediate relief. They do not daily witness their patients recovering from illnesses like measles or mumps under the guidance of Nature alone.

Animals have no doctors; they rely solely on Nature to heal them. If an animal in the wild breaks a leg, it seeks shelter and refuses food, drinking only water if it can get it, until Nature achieves a recovery. Drugs play no part in the animal's recovery, yet animals can heal perfectly, given the chance.

Were doctors – and patients – to witness just a few cases in which drugs were not used yet full recovery was made, they would surely be converted.

Medical doctors, such as those who practise the Gerson Therapy, who witness full recoveries by diet alone, are a privileged minority. The average doctor would probably consider any colleague who relied on Nature to do the healing as a crank – and that has happened to many a good physician.

Shunned

Dr. Richard Mackarness, who brought the concept of food and chemical allergies to Britain in the mid-1970s, had tremendous successes with previously 'intractable' conditions. As a psychiatrist, he applied the food allergy approach to his mental patients with considerable success, but paid the price for it by being shunned by former colleagues who could not match his success record.

He was able to restore to sanity several very seriously mentally ill patients. One such lady was being considered for brain surgery when he, in a meeting of psychiatrists in the Park Prewett Psychiatric hospital in Basingstoke, suggested he try, for the first time in Britain, the food/chemical allergy approach. Considering they had nothing to lose, they allowed Mackarness to use the approach, one that they probably considered futile.

So remarkable was the lady's recovery that not only was her brain operation cancelled, but she returned home to look after her children successfully, only becoming ill again whenever she broke her diet.

His doctor colleagues, probably embarrassed that they had failed to identify such an obvious causative factor as diet, slowly ostracised him and he eventually went to live in Australia. This practice of shunning fellow doctors who stray from the 'straight and narrow' is extremely common.

In the middle of the last century, Prof. Austin Flint, one of the most prominent American physicians of his day, cared for a large number of cases of pneumonia without drugs of any kind and without a single death. About the same time another prominent New York physician cared for a number of cases of typhus without drugs, again without losing a patient. The city's Academy of Medicine voted to take the matter up for discussion at its next meeting but the discussion was never held. It would have been extremely embarrassing to the medical profession and financially crippling to the wealthy drug companies to openly admit that these seemingly dangerous conditions could recover of their own accord, without any drugs whatsoever, by leaving healing to the body's powerful innate ability.

Oliver Wendell Holmes was a revered Professor of Anatomy and Physiology at Harvard Medical School for 35 years. It is little wonder that he was ostricised by the medical profession when he openly declared that if all the drugs in the world were cast into the sea, it would be the better for mankind and the worse for the fishes.

All drugs are poisons; it is only a matter of degree

Drugs enter the bloodstream and are carried by this means to every organ and tissue in the body. The bloodstream bathes all parts of the body with its contents. If it carries drugs, which are poisonous, then these poisons touch every aspect of our system.

Not all drugs are eliminated by the body; residues build up within our systems and no-one can be sure what adverse influence these poisons may have on our long-term health. No matter what tests are carried out on animals prior to a drug getting a 'safe' tag so that it can be made available to humans, no long term testing on humans is done – until that is, the drug reaches the general marketplace.

We may be able to witness a side-effect of some drugs that manifest as say, a rash, because this is visible. A drug's other likely influences may lie deep within the system – out of sight – and so can only be measured in guesswork terms.

How many chronic sufferers are there in this country today who are maintaining their diseased state by treating themselves with the very drugs that are prolonging their disease, or have, indeed, caused further medical complications? The taking of drugs can prevent healing in many cases. If the condition had been left alone in the first place, more often than not true healing would have been accomplished by the body itself and Nature would have been allowed to show off her own healing skills, particularly if improved diet had been adopted.

To create a condition of ill health through many years of eating a poor or artificial diet and then to seek to remedy that condition by taking drugs whilst continuing to consume the very cause of your ill health, is foolhardy.

Vaccinations and cot-deaths

Vaccinations commonly used throughout the world have taken on a mantle of efficacy that is ill deserved. Many so-called epidemics appear around the globe in up-and-down patterns, with or without the peoples being vaccinated.

These epidemics (or pandemics) disappear of their own accord. The influence of vaccinations in their disappearance is questionable. Many books decrying the entire vaccination system have been published, most of them indicating that vast sums of money are at the root of it all. I quote from the Gerson Healing Newsletter of August 1997:

> We have long been acutely aware of the dangers of infant vaccinations and plan on doing a longer article about it in the near future. In the meantime, I should like to make our readers aware of a report reproduced in the British Gerson Support Group's publication of June 1996: In one publication Dr. Viera Scheibner, ('Vaccination') states the following: 'The diphtheria, pertussis (whooping cough) and tetanus (DPT) vaccine is given to babies as young as six to eight weeks old in many countries – including the USA. It is implicated in many cases of cot death. Interestingly, in Japan in 1975 the vaccination age was moved to the age of two, and cot death disappeared.

Diagnosis

I sincerely hope that the reader of this book does not consider I am entirely decrying the medical profession: its ability to diagnose serious illness and thereby provide peace of mind to a worried mum with a sick child is undoubtedly a great service. However, more attention should be given to what is already known by the medical profession: Nature and Nature alone heals, not the doctor!

Surgeons, too, can often perform work that unquestionably saves lives, especially after accidents, or in such fine cases as the separation of Siamese Twins. But surgery is often over-used and many operations have been cancelled after a patient has sought dietary help for their condition.

At one time arthritis sufferers were advised to change climates, were given hot baths, sulfa baths, massages and diathermy treatments, whilst every conceivable (known) dietetic novelty was freely tried. Then, the theory came in that not only rheumatoid arthritis, rheumatic fever and rheumatic heart were to be conquered by the use of hormones, but it was even hoped that the answer to the overall cancer problem and many of the other diseases of man may be found in hormone research. Cortisone and ACTH grew out of hormone research. Not only their failure but also their devastating effects are now universally admitted.

Many modes of treatment for arthritis have been in vogue at different times. Searching through the literature produced over just a few decades will unearth a bewildering array of drugs that were used in the treatment of arthritis. Bleeding, local and general, together with other so-called anti-inflammatory measures, were extensively used. Mercury was given to the point of salivation, and colchicum in order to make the patient vomit; an ounce or more daily of nitrate of potash, opium in full doses, and other drugs were in vogue during the twenty-five year period prior to 1863. In the 1860s the method generally adopted consisted of salts of pottassa or soda in sufficient quantity to render the urine alkaline. This was known as the 'alkaline treatment'.

Suffice it to say that any review of these treatments reveals that, although many may have had certain palliative powers, the results obtained under each and every one, the duration of the disease, the tendency to develop other concomitant conditions including nervous diseases, pulmonary troubles, digestive disorders, diseases of the urinary organs etc., all indicate that none of them was of any value whatsoever in removing the condition permanently. None of the treatments tackled or sought the cause. Indeed, there is every evidence to believe that most of the complications and concomitant ailments were directly due to the treatments given to these patients.

Yet the number of recoveries from arthritis that are achieved by 'merely' altering the patients' diets is ever increasing, as more and more people are taught that it is the abuse of their bodies by long term, unnatural dietary choices that is the actual cause of this painful disease. So long as the condition has not reached the stage of being irreversible, there is hope for the arthritis sufferer if he only will listen to, and apply, the correct dietary advice.

Evidence continues to mount that poor 'Western' diets are at the root of much of our modern illnesses. Heart disease in Japan is very low even today in comparison to the U.S.A. and studies have shown that when a Japanese person goes to live in the U.S.A. and starts to eat the awful American diet of burgers, coke and suchlike, he too will succumb to the dreadful killer. Those Japanese who maintain their Japanese diets in the U.S.A. are spared the disease! Americans may lead the world in technological advancements but they have gone too far in one area, and that is the 'advancement' of what should never be interfered with by man, our diet. The introduction of fast foods, junk foods, T.V. dinners and the like, may suit the palates of present-day youngsters, but ill health awaits them as a result.

There is more than enough evidence to show that drugs, despite being declared 'safe' for your doctor to prescribe, can cause you considerable harm – even death.

Dr. Vernon Coleman, himself medically trained, writing in the *Journal of Alternative and Complementary* Medicine, July 1994, stated that it was estimated that over one million patients are in hospital beds in the U.K. as a direct result of iatrogenesis – damage caused by (prescribed) drug taking.

Make no mistake about it, the ordinary tablets given to you by your doctor could, over a period of time, greatly affect your health for the worse. Although these drugs are passed as 'safe' by the powerful pharmaceutical companies, it is often only a matter of time before they are taken off the market again because they are shown to have ominous long-term effects, many very serious indeed.

Shelton observed that an estimated 85% of the drugs now in use were unknown 25 years ago. All of them, however brief their period of popularity, leave an aftermath of trouble in their wake. In spite of this failure to find drugs that 'cure', the search goes on night and day throughout the world for the magic bullet for this or that ailment.

Hardly a day goes by without a newspaper somewhere announcing a new wonder drug to cure cancer or heart disease, when the evidence is mountainous that these two conditions are caused by inappropriate diet. If the cause of an illness is poor diet, how can continuing the diet but eating a drug on top remove the cause of that illness? To remove the actual cause you have to, like it or not, change your eating habits.

The rise and fall of new drugs follows a common enough pattern.[125] Firstly, there is the discovery of the drug, followed by sensational announcements of its claims in the press and television. These claims are more often than not simply what is *projected* as likely to happen in the future, in other words what wonderful benefits the drug will have in restoring us to health.

Secondly, there follows the marketing and employment of the new drug with overly-optimistic forecasts of the cures the new drug is about to perform.

Thirdly, there follows a period of comparative silence, during which the drug is widely used in a wide variety of symptom complexes.

Fourthly, there follows notification of the side effects of this drug, together with the usual warning about these 'adverse reactions.'

Finally, the drugs falls into disuse, as another new discovery takes its place, to follow the same course of promise, hope, expectancy and inevitable failure.

Scientists and doctors around the world are searching for new drugs that can make them rich beyond their wildest dreams. The Nature Cure approach to healing holds no riches for anyone. There is little money to be made from it. Only, as Gerson remarked, the greengrocer, would benefit.

Dr. Herbert Shelton would fast patients before putting them onto 'Hygienic' diets (essentially Nature Cure diets consisting of mostly fruits and vegetables), achieving remarkable results during his lifetime. Lengthy fasts of 30 and upwards days were considered quite normal and he achieved what many doctors would consider impossible in the way of recoveries from serious or long-standing illnesses.

Shelton recalls an autopsy which was performed on a three-year-old girl in San Antonio in Texas. The child had been taken to the hospital the evening before and found to be dead upon arrival. According to the father, the child was given a 'dose of medicine' on the first morning of the 'treatment of a cold'. During the day she became violently ill. When he returned home in the evening the child collapsed and was dead before he could get her to the hospital.

Children, Shelton observed, do not die of colds. They do not sicken in the morning and die suddenly in the evening of the same day of a cold.

Whatever the autopsy finding may have been, we can be sure that this child died of the 'cure'. Whether she received the 'wrong' medicine or an overdose of the 'right' medicine, she died of drug poisoning. The violent illness that developed after the 'remedy' was administered was the violent efforts of the little organism to rid itself of the poison.

Shelton explained: each and every one of us should realise that the only drugs in all the chemists in the land that are properly labelled are those labelled with the skull and crossbones. There is no such thing as a non-poisonous drug. Some are of greater virulence than others, but all are poisonous.

Shelton recalls in his own words in his *Hygienic Review* of April 1968 the following story which pays tribute to the power of the human organism's healing efforts whilst fasting:

'My baby is dying.' These plaintive words of a despairing mother came to me over the telephone in the early morning one day in the winter of 1927 or 1928. (My records have been destroyed and an exact date is not possible.)

I was living in New York at the time and was on the staff of the Macfadden publications, writing for *Physical Culture* and other publications of that organization. I had a daily column in the *New York Graphic* and feature articles in the magazine section of the Graphic on occasion. The woman identified herself as Mrs Marvin Hall of Nyack, New York. I did not know Mrs Hall and she did not know me. She had been reading my articles in the Graphic and appealed to me in her distress.

I asked her: 'How do you know that your baby is dying, Mrs Hall?' She replied: 'My baby has pneumonia and a consultation of four physicians has just rendered this verdict. They say there is nothing more that they can do, that the baby will die.'

I said to Mrs Hall: 'Let's fool them!' She replied: 'That is exactly what I want to do. I want my baby to live.'

I said: 'Mrs Hall, listen carefully and follow these instructions exactly. Go to the bedside of your baby and sweep all that mass of drugs on the table by its bed into the waste basket and see that the baby does not get another dose of drugs. Open the window and let some fresh air into the room. Keep the baby warm. Give it no food. Give it water according to thirst. Report to me tomorrow morning.'

Each morning for the next few mornings, Mrs Hall called me on the telephone and reported the daily progress of her baby. The progress was much faster than we could have hoped for and the baby's recovery was soon complete. About 20 years passed and Madelyn Hall (the baby's name), now grown into a lovely young lady, was married.

21.

The Path to Recovery

If we take take on board all the evidence that we have come across thus far: the Pottenger's Cats experiments showing how critical to health proper diet is, not only to the adult but the offspring as well; the Hunza diet, responsible for superb health amongst these peoples – and proven by replicating the diet in mice; the evidence of the Gerson Therapy, remedying all manner of previously-considered-intractable disease; the evidence that low body temperature can produce many symptoms of ill health and that body temperature can *rise* by applying a diet of mostly natural foods, then we are left with only one valid conclusion, and that is, if we intend to recover our health, the nutritional approach can be the only answer.

The Nature Cure approach is simply another way of saying you are eating as Nature intended. That is how many thousands of people have recovered their health and such an approach is what the food/chemical allergic patient, and anyone who has any sort of chronic illness, should adopt.

If you consider that by applying a natural dietary approach you are 'merely' improving your diet, then common sense must tell you that it cannot be harmful. You should be aware of this, lest well-meaning friends and relatives suggest you are doing something wrong. Simply ask anyone who suggests your changed eating pattern might cause you problems: 'How on earth can improving your diet be harmful?'.

People tend to be afraid of the unfamiliar, and as 'natural eating' is so different from the usual diet in developed countries, then they may well voice genuine if unfounded fears. Such fears will often be heard during flare-ups, when you may appear to become worse, so warn your friends, if you must, that these 'crises' are Nature's method of cleansing the system, not harming it.

Although it may prove quite difficult for many such sufferers to dramatically alter their eating habits, if their suffering is sufficiently incapacitating, then they have little option other but to apply this approach. At least, with this new information, you will be able to monitor your progress as no-one has done before, by charting your daily temperature and recognising that slowly – and surely – your vitality, along with your temperature, will be increasing! The dietary means by which recovery can be achieved not only dictates what you put into your mouth, but, just as importantly, what you don't.

A complete turn-around of the dietary failings which brought about your illness in the first place is essential. Assuming there was a period in your life when your present condition did not exist, then the only means of restoring your health to that of a 'pre-food-allergy-condition' or a 'pre-illness-condition' is by totally – not partially – reversing the poor eating habits that derailed your health.

The build-up of unwanted deposits in your blood vessels and connective tissues around the body has to be eroded away. This build-up, which will almost certainly exist around your many thousands of miles of tiny arteries and veins, will have gone a long way to reducing your vitality and thereby laying the unhealthy 'soil' that is so suitable to parasite habitation.

As the unwanted build-up of deposits will have taken place over a long time, because of poor dietary choice, the very same means – dietary – can be employed to slowly reverse it. This same dietary approach will help restore health to areas in your body that require regeneration, such as damaged or unhealthy tissue.

Recovery by diet takes time, although you should see hopeful early signs within a short time, sometimes days. Some people take longer to recover than others. Often this is dependent upon how much previous medication has been taken by the patient. The more drugged the individual has been in the past, the longer it often takes for such a person to achieve full recovery. That is not a hard and fast rule, so do not be despondent about your previous drug taking – it simply takes time for drugs to be eliminated from the system.

By turning around your eating habits you can reverse, at least to a great extent, your present state of health. How far this reversal goes depends on a number of things: the length of time you have been with symptoms, what the actual symptoms are, how seriously deficient your previous diet was, how much drugging has taken place in the past, how rigidly you stick to the advice given, and the length of time you now adhere to the new diet.

Nature Cure establishments and fasting experts are always loathe to say that any condition is irreversible, for they are constantly coming across conditions, considered irreversible, which in fact do reverse. If the patient stops the diet early, whether due to lack of willpower or any other reason, then no-one will be able to know just what improvement might have been waiting round the corner.

If there is a family history of your condition, it is wrong to worry yourself sick that there is no hope. There have been hundreds of cases where the 'hereditary condition' has been foiled and the patient does not fall victim to it.

Remember that, if you do nothing, then if you are going to get it, you are going to get it. But if you tackle the condition by enormously improving your diet, that can only help your health. Read the chapter on hereditary illness for encouragement: you DO have more control than you thought!

There is documented evidence of so-called hereditary conditions being avoided and even reversed by applying natural eating methods. The Gerson therapy twins who were 'born with' Takayasu's disease – the so–called 'pulse-less disease' – were able to restore themselves to health simply by improving their diet. Do not therefore despair if your parents had total disregard for their own diets, as it is still possible to remedy your own bodily condition.

The food allergic

The food allergic attempting to restore health by applying a natural diet may well be faced with a special problem. He may well find that items on the diet, even although they may be organically grown, can provoke an 'allergic' response. Your symptoms can flare up despite eating what are normally considered to be 'healing foods'.

Ideally, one should avoid all allergens. However, as is frequently the case, natural-food diets may be top-heavy in foods that provoke symptoms. Remember of course that we should not blame the foods – we have already explained that it is the food allergic's body that is at fault and not the natural foods.

If you are a food allergic consuming food allergens whilst on such a recovery programme, there are two ways of handling the situation. One is to avoid food allergens at all cost, by which you may compromise the actual course of the therapy through sheer reduction of quality – and quantity – of incoming nutrients.

The other way is effectively to say 'To hell with my allergies' and just eat foods to which you know you are 'allergic'! This may sound absurd advice but there is a logic to it. Countless patients through the years have restored themselves to full health by dietary means, whether the 'old-fashioned' Nature Cure approach available in such-styled establishments, or other diets such as the Gerson. Although these diets might have been applied to conquer a life-threatening condition, patients would often also have secondary complaints which were not life-threatening but which were still capable of making their life miserable; arthritis is a good example.

Very often these patients would get a double bonus: their main illness would clear up and they would find that their other symptoms had too.

Now, as most food allergic patients will know, arthritis is one extremely common food allergy condition that can be influenced by many dietary substances. The food connection to arthritis is so common as to be almost compulsory! It is still the case, however, that very many arthritis sufferers are unfamiliar with testing for food or chemical allergies and bear their lot without knowing of the food link.

It therefore follows that many patients following the Gerson diet will not have been routinely tested for food allergies and indeed, will not even know of any possible food link; they nevertheless find their arthritis clearing up regardless, just by staying on the diet. So, by disregarding the food allergy link and adhering for a sustained period of time to the diet, they still made a full recovery.

There is another common sense manner in which to view this phenomenon. There are many 'universal reactors': food allergic patients who react to virtually every food or drink that they encounter. There is nothing they can eat or drink which does not provoke a response.

Logically therefore, one has to realise there can only be three possible options open to such a patient:

(i) Stop eating and drinking altogether and thus avoid all contact with allergenic foodstuffs.
    or
(ii) Ignore the food allergy angle entirely and simply eat one's old diet (the diet that led to the trouble in the first place).
    or
(iii) Ignore the food allergy angle entirely and dramatically raise the nutritional status of one's diet to one that bears no semblance to the old diet that produced the ill-health in the first place.

If you accept that the first option, to stop eating and drinking, would be foolish, then there are only two options left.

To carry on eating as we did before would be pointless, as this was responsible for bringing about the condition in the first place. Eating in this way has not removed the condition so why persevere?

The third option is the only one left: dramatically to turn around one's diet to one that has a proven history of restoring health – the Nature Cure approach. There is a strong possibility that one will still be consuming foods which may provoke a response. But the overall nutrition is entirely different to what was previously eaten, and it is this which will be the saviour of the patient who takes this option. It is this improved nutrition that will raise the body temperature to bring about the health recovery.

But how can it be that one can eat food allergens and still get well? The following analogy will suffice to explain the phenomenon. Imagine for a moment that you had toothache or a gum infection, which was so sore that you could hardly eat. Then assume that you tried to eat an organically grown apple.

Of course, it would hurt. But undoubtedly the food would be good for your body. If you did manage to eat the apple, say by chewing on the good side of your mouth, it would ultimately add to your overall nutritional status. The nutrients supplied by the apple would course through the bloodstream, bathing every tissue and organ in the body, including the troublesome gum or tooth area. So you would be eating something that might cause temporary pain in your body, but at the same time indirectly restoring overall health to your system.

So too with the arthritis sufferer (with a food allergy connection to his illness) who takes a natural diet approach. He might temporarily be aggravating his arthritis or any other condition linked to food allergy by virtue of eating food allergens, but if he continues eating this way — which is a vast improvement over his old artificial diet — his body will relish the improved nutrition and consequently respond by restoring health to all parts of his body, including the area that shows arthritis; the area that is the site of his food allergy reactions.

As the overall nutrition of the body improves, so too will its healing abilities, which depend on proper nutrition to function. These healing powers at work are effectively the restoration of areas around the body that require normalising, whether removing unnatural deposits in blood vessels (which may make the area attractive to parasites), or correcting true nutritional deficiencies like scurvy. But these healing powers also restore health by making the body's own eliminatory powers more effective, ridding the system of undesirable toxins and generally achieving a long-needed cleansing of the entire system.

Progress

The progress that can be expected as the diet goes on and the body temperature increases, is that any symptom normally considered a 'food allergic' symptom will reduce in intensity. Any reactions will gradually reduce in severity.

There will be flare-ups when the symptoms may get apparently worse, but this will be followed by periods of reduced intensity. There will be many ups and downs, but the overall pattern will be of a reduction in severity and duration, until eventually the symptoms — the food allergy — will be no longer! You will witness a correlation between the erratic nature of the body temperature increases and the erratic nature of your symptom improvement. Once the temperature rises, and *stabilises*, you will see a lasting improvement in your condition.

Withdrawal symptoms

Withdrawal symptoms are a feature of Nature Cure diets just as they are with other 'ordinary' dietary programmes. The giving up of your previous stimulants and addictions will result in a period of feeling miserable.

As you are 'coming off' your old diet, almost certainly top heavy in addictive substances such as coffee or bread, withdrawal symptoms of headache, fatigue, depression and various aches and pains will undoubtedly appear. These shouldn't last for more than 2 or 3 days after which you should feel considerably better. But, miserable though they may be, they should be recognised as a sign of improvement: your body is shaking itself free of an addictive and toxic load and that is a step forward, towards health.

As the weeks go on, you may experience a 'healing crisis', which may incorporate a fever. The raised temperature may also exist alongside other vague symptoms of distress. Under no circumstances should efforts be made to interfere with the course of the fever. Drugs must NOT be taken as, at such a time, they could be dangerous (see my discussion on fever elsewhere in this book). Nature, if given the chance, will guide your body to recovery, safely and definitely. Your body will be all the better for having gone through the fever, which is Nature's way of speeding up the elimination of old toxins. A fever during a Nature Cure dietary regimen should not be feared, but welcomed with open arms.

Such a healing fever can occur at any time during the recovery programme you will undertake, but most commonly after a month or so of such treatment. It can recur throughout the long road to recovery, appearing every month or six weeks or so, reminding the patient that there is indeed activity going on within his body. Individuals vary, and there can be no strict period set down in advance as to when one can expect a healing crisis. Nor can the manner or duration of the crisis be forecast.

Beata Bishop, in her book *A Time to Heal* observed the oddity of the fact that, at the Gerson clinic, patients would eagerly seek the onset of a fever, so much so that they would ask each other if they had had one yet. The healing crisis was considered almost a badge of honour and you weren't a 'proper' Gerson patient until you had experienced one! In the 'outside world' however, anyone with a fever would be probably rushed to hospital where great efforts would be made to reduce it.

Such intervention would be considered outrageous – indeed even dangerous – by anyone knowledgeable in natural healing. To interrupt Nature's effort in restoring health – the fever – can be dangerous. At best it will set back the organism's attempts to remedy the condition. You must persevere with the diet and not imagine that a fever means the diet is not working.

22.

The Recovery Programme

We can quite readily achieve relief from our symptom merely by identifying our food allergens and thereafter avoiding them. But to achieve full and total recovery from our illness – and that includes the actual food allergy syndrome itself so that you no longer react to foods – a SUSTAINED period on natural foods is required. This may take from 9 months to a year, or in some cases up to 2 or even 3 years, depending upon a number of factors such as

(i)   How long you have been ill

(ii) How long your temperature has been abnormal

(iii) The quality of your former diet

(iv) How much medication/alcohol/tobacco has previously been consumed

(v)   Your ability to respond (everybody will respond, but some will take longer than others)

Remember, there will be many periods during the recovery programme when you may well feel worse. This is to be expected, so do not let it put you off.

Take your morning underarm temperature, whilst in bed before you rise or become active, and mark it in a diary. Take it for a full ten minutes. The supposed range indicative of reasonable health, according to Dr. Broda Barnes, is 97.8-98.2F. The figure of 98.6F. however is the accepted temperature indicating normal health in man.

Perhaps we have reduced our sights over the past few decades as our health has slumped? We should be looking to increase our temperature, certainly out of the danger zone, which is below 97.80, preferably to above 98.2F.

Keep recording your morning temperature using the ten minute method. If practicable, try and take a mid afternoon temperature reading as well. You need only take a five minute reading at this time of day, and taking the temperature under the tongue will suffice. Even if your morning temperature does not reach 98.6 degrees F., your afternoon one may on occasion, showing that progress is being made.

At the end of each month make up a graph of the month's readings. By keeping such records you will be recording definite *evidence* that your new diet is working. If you do not keep such a record, the erratic nature of the improvement and the slowness of natural cure might well dishearten you. Seeing the improved temperature readings in black and white will do wonders for morale!

When your symptoms disappear, there may be a tendency to slacken off your diet. It is important to *maintain* the practice of recording your daily temperatures. If your temperature starts to slip back, remedy it by a return to dietary intensification.

The likely pattern will be one of erratic temperatures at first ,then *stabilising* at the higher figures. When that happens, most improvement will be seen. The longer you maintain stable temperatures, the less likelihood there is of you falling ill again. To use someone else's expression, the further you are in the bed, the less likely you are to fall out!

Duration

It is simply not possible to state at the outset how long one needs to stay on this fairly strict dietary regimen until recovery is complete. Everyone is different, with varying degrees of toxicity, symptoms, past drug or alcohol excesses and ability to respond to improved nutrition. Some people take longerthan others. But watching your body temperature improve as the weeks go by will be the most important indicator that your health is improving!

Once your body temperature increases and you *sustain* this increase for a time, your symptoms will decrease and ultimately disappear. No one, as I state, can put a time on this, but what is important is that your higher body temperature is sustained to ensure that any parasites you do have will be well and truly inactivated or destroyed.

If you return too quickly to your old, health-destroying diet, then your body temperature will eventually drop; It is up to you to maintain it at a high level and thus defeat your symptoms.

Once your temperature has been raised to the limits that your body can achieve (and no-one is able to predict what that will be in any one person; you have to watch the progress of your temperatures to determine this) and you have gone some time without symptoms, you can then afford yourself the luxury of an occasional night out. Such a treat will not seriously interfere with your body temperature as long as, firstly, you have reached your maximum body temperature and sustained it for a good period to stabilise your health, and secondly, the occasional night out does not turn into a five-day-a-week round of binges! However, keep the graph going so you are forever alert to any drop back in temperature.

The diet might seem very restrictive, certainly in comparison to the freedom of choice you might have thus far enjoyed, but you will soon get into the swing of things and the feeling of deprivation truly will disappear.

Once you start experimenting with delicious home-made soups, it will become a relative joy. And when you see what it does for your body temperature over the first 3 or 4 months, you will have definitive proof that something is happening inside you, something that can have only one possible implication:

YOUR HEALTH IS RETURNING

Good luck!

Recovery Programme

The following diet should be followed for at least a year. Some people will need to adhere to it for twice that time, others less; no-one can predict. But your personal temperature graph will be best indicator of all – do not relax it.

IMPORTANT NOTES

(1) **If you are a food allergic who reacts to many foods on this regimen read the last chapter, which explains you can still get well by perseverance. You can, if you only have a few food allergies, avoid the foods that affect you: the choice is yours.**

(2) **Asthmatics, epilepsy sufferers, and patients with serious psychiatric symptoms should only pursue the following diet under the guidance of a naturopath, clinical ecologist, nutritional therapist, a knowledgeable doctor, or someone experienced in Nature Cure dietary approaches and food/chemical allergies, as symptoms can worsen at times, before improving, during the course of the diet.**

(3) To get the full benefit of the diet, all drugs should be tapered off and eventually stopped. This however should not be done alone; but under the guidance of your doctor.

(4) To get the full benefit of the diet, you must stop smoking!

All fruits and vegetables should ideally be organically grown. If you choose to eat foods that have been sprayed with pesticides, this will add to your toxic load, when the very object of this diet is to raise your body temperature by flushing out old deposits. Recovery will take longer if you choose to eat foods contaminated with these sprays. Do not eat anything tinned or packaged as the valuable enzymes will almost certainly have been destroyed.

Raw foods

Rawness is critical: you must have raw food at least once a day, either as a raw mixed salad (perhaps with a baked potato) or as fruits such as oranges or pears. The more raw the content of your diet, the faster your body will respond.

Foods allowed

All fruits, especially:

PEACHES • ORANGES
APRICOTS • APPLES
PLUMS • PEARS
BANANAS • AVOCADO
GRAPES • MELONS
TOMATOES • CHERRIES

Fruit and Vegetable Juices:

Excellent and freely allowed if the machine you use is one that triturates (grinds) and not one that works by centrifugal force. The grinding machine (such as the Champion or Norwalk) can be very expensive. If you do not have such a machine, you can still use an ordinary juicer as a compromise, but it *may* slow the process.

Vegetable juices are thoroughly recommended and you should aim for an absolute minimum of six 8oz glasses per day. The Gerson Therapy recommends 13 glasses, spread over the day at hourly intervals and if you can manage that, then all the better, most especially during the first six months of the diet. Do *not* drink juices from cartons, bottles or cans, no matter how 'natural' the advertising suggests it is; they will undoubtedly have been heated at some stage on their journey to the shop and such heating destroys the enzymes and vitamins.

Vegetables

All vegetables can be used, including potatoes (boiled or baked in their skins only). If you find you are putting on weight (you will not necessarily do so) cut down on potatoes.

Soups

Two or three bowls a day. Make your own. Use organically grown vegetables and pulses that you can buy from your wholefood shop. You can make an excellent soup using *no stock* whatsoever. I suggest the following simply to show you that a tasty soup can be achieved without the addition of artificial stocks or meats.

CARROTS, POT BARLEY, ONIONS, GREEN SPLIT PEAS, GARLIC, YELLOW SPLIT PEAS, BROCCOLI, RED SPLIT LENTILS, LEEKS, CABBAGE, GREEN LENTILS.

Chop the vegetables roughly and bring to the boil in sufficient water to cover them. Simmer for one hour, then serve.

You can add other vegetables to the above to suit your taste such as cauliflower or turnip; experiment to find your own favourite.

Salads

Eat at least one large, raw salad each day, and snacks of fruit. The salads can be composed of some fruits and any vegetables, finely grated if required, such as

LEEK, CARROTS, BOILED POTATO, BEETROOT, LETTUCE, BROCCOLI, CAULIFLOWER, TOMATOES, CELERY, GREEN/ RED/YELLOW PEPPERS, CUCUMBER, MIXED BEAN SPROUTS, GARLIC, SPROUTED MUNG BEANS, ONIONS, NUTS (once a week), APPLES, BANANAS, PEAR SLICES

Grains

Oatmeal; preferably organic wholegrain, as porridge. Can be taken if desired, on a daily basis. Do not add milk. You can add sliced banana if desired.

Wholemeal bread: get organic if possible. One or two slices a day allowed. It is best not to eat bread until month three, as even organic bread contains salt, which you should avoid!

After 1 month the following can be added (if desired):

WHITE FISH: once a week
UNSALTED BUTTER: organic, sparingly.

After 3 months the following can be added (if desired):

FREE RANGE EGGS: no more than two per week

After 6 months the following can be added (if desired):

RAW (UNPASTEURISED) MILK: no more than one cup per week

Not allowed

SALT (table, and in processed foods), PACKAGED FRUIT JUICES, MILK, ALCOHOL, SALTED BUTTER, TOBACCO, CHEESE, WHITE FLOUR, MEAT, COFFEE, WHITE RICE, TEA, WHITE BREAD, CAKES, FLUORIDE TOOTHPASTES, CHOCOLATES, CREAM, ICE CREAM, CANNED BEVERAGES, SUGAR, FAT, TINNED, FROZEN AND PACKAGED FOODS,

The preceeding list of forbidden substances is not exhaustive. Use common sense and do not consume anything that comes pre-packed or processed.

Cooking Utensils

Use stainless steel if possible. Do not use aluminium pots or pans as the aluminium can leach into the cooking water.

Note: the above is not the strict version of the Gerson therapy but a variation of it. The version given in this programme was the one followed by the author and which achieved the temperature increase.

The stricter Gerson therapy, with 13 glasses of organic raw vegetable and fruit juices each day as well as some medications will undoubtedly achieve the same result and probably quicker. If you wish to follow the Gerson therapy fully, details are available from the Gerson Institute, the address of which is given in the address section at the end of this book

23.

How Man Should Eat

There have been many arguments, even among nutritionists, as to whether man is a carnivore, omnivore, a herbivore or a frugivore. To settle the argument, one need only look at the gastrointestinal and dental make-up of various species. If you compare the anthropoid ape with man anatomically and physiologically you will see the striking similarities.

It would make sound common sense that Nature would make our intended diet one that we would seek out; one that we would relish. I consider man would not readily seek out cold, hard, turnips in the ground, almost certainly heavily caked in soil; no matter how delicious they may taste in soups. I would suspect that the design of Nature would be that we would be attracted to foods by their smell and hence, their taste. The taste of raw turnip would hardly attract primitive man, I should think.

Rather it is my view that man would seek out, in the wild, ripe juicy fruits such as pears, plums, melons, oranges, apples etc., which would make us frugivores. As the ape also subsists on this diet, with the addition of some nuts, we could reasonably say that man is intended to eat in like manner, given that man and ape's anatomy and physiology are virtually identical.

All the evidence in Nature Cure, the Hunza diet, Pottenger's Cats experiments and Weston Price's observations are that the diet of man would produce best health if there was a preponderance of raw fruits in it.

As I have stated elsewhere, humans do not need to eat meat in order to build muscle. The huge bulk of the rhinoceros, the enormous power of the ape, the massive frame of the bull; the colossus that is the elephant – all are testament to the fact that huge musculature can be built up by fruit and grasses alone.

Nature has certainly given us the ability to cope with food choices other than fruits, doubtless as a means of survival in times of famine, but I feel that for maximum health and freedom from disease, we should be guided by the make-up of our digestive systems and eat accordingly. As suggested in the following comparisons, I propose that man is intended to eat in the manner of the ape, viz: fruits and nuts.

CHAPTER TWENTY-THREE

Is man carnivore, omnivore, herbivore or frugivore?

	Carnivores	Omnivores
Placenta	Zonary	non-deciduate
Limbs	Four-footed	Four-footed
	Have claws	Have hoofs
Locomotion	On all fours	On all fours
	Tails	Tails
Eye direction	Look sideways	Look sideways
Skin pores	Without	With
Incisor teeth	Slightly developed	Very well developed
Molar teeth	Pointed	In folds
Dental Formula★	5 to 8.1.6.1.5 to 8 5 to 8.1.6.1.5 to 8	8.1.2 to 3.1.8 8.1.2 to 3.1.8
Salivary glands	Small	Well developed
Saliva & Urine	Acid reaction	Acid
Tongue	Rasping	Smooth
Teats/Mammaries	On abdomen	On abdomen
Stomach	Simple and roundish,	Simple and roundish, large cul-de-sac
Intestinal canal size	3 times legnth of body	10 times length of body
Intestinal canal	Smooth colon	Smooth & convoluted
Diet	Flesh	Flesh, carrion & plants

★ The figures in the centre represent the number of incisors, on each side are the canines, followed to the left and right are the mollars.

Herbivores	Anthropoid Apes	Man
non–deciduate	Discoidal	Discoidal
Four-footed	2 hands & 2 feet	2 hands & 2 feet
Cloven hoofs	Flat nails	Flat nails
On all fours	Walks upright	Walks upright
Tails	Without tails	Without tails
Look sideways	Look forward	Look forward
With	Millions	Millions
None	Well developed	Well developed
None	Blunt	Blunt
6.0.0.0.6 6.1.6.1.6	5.1.4.1.5 5.1.4.1.5	5.1.4.1.5 5.1.4.1.5
Well developed	Well developed	Well developed
Alkaline	Alkaline	Alkaline
Smooth	Smooth	Smooth
On abdomen	On breast	On breast
3 compartments, 4 in camels & some ruminents	One, with duodenum as second stomach	One, with duodenum as second stomach
Species vary but usually 10 times legnth of body	12 times legnth of body	12 times legnth of body
Smooth & convoluted	Colon convoluted	Colon convoluted
Grass, herbs & plants	Fruits & nuts	Fruits & nuts

24.

The Food Allergy Conundrum

It is becoming clear that virtually any symptom of ill health can have a food link. Many articles in newspapers and magazines over recent years have referred to 'food allergies' as being responsible for a host of common disorders and, as a result, more and more people are finding the connection themselves. Not only foods, but drinks, inhalants and indeed even chemicals found around the house are showing to be responsible for many common symptoms.

The term 'food allergy' in this context is a misnomer, at least as far as conventional allergists are concerned.

'Classical' allergists tend not to be interested in the masked food allergy condition, which is what this book is about. Those who are interested often do not have the time or indeed the know-how to identify accurately the culprit foods, for it can indeed be time consuming. The hospital allergist who is confronted by a patient claiming food allergy will have a limited number of methods at his or her disposal to attempt the diagnosis and what is available is often inappropriate. The commonly-applied skin tests are notoriously unreliable indicators of food allergies.

The word allergy was not coined until 1906. The early allergists would concern themselves mostly with the obvious manifestations of illnesses such as hay fever, apparently caused by airborne proteins such as pollen. The 'aeroallergen' (inhalant) aspect of allergies was far more considered than foodstuffs. Or they would study the reactions in laboratory animals to such seemingly innocent substances as serums and egg white. The hay fever and any adverse reactions in the animals would be put down to the operation of the immune system. This is the system that enables us to fight off bacteria and causes the body to reject, say, a skin graft supplied by another person. As Dr. Ben Feingold states:

Allergy cannot be defined without a consideration of the nature of immunity. Immunity involves all the mechanisms concerned with the protection of the individual against the assault of foreign substances. A foreign substance is any material which the body does not recognise as self, i.e., a part of itself…

Since allergy is a variation of the basic immune mechanism, a discussion of allergy is actually a consideration of the mechanism of immunity.[126]

The body recognises pollen as being 'foreign' to it; yet conventional allergists do not appear to have considered just why everybody exposed to pollen does not have a hay fever reaction.

Everyday foods are now recognised as being responsible for symptoms of ill health, but as these are not considered 'foreign' to the body, conventional allergists are reluctant to accept the food allergy phenomenon as being widespread, though it undoubtedly is.

Immunological

By 1926, the descriptive term 'allergy' was redefined immunologically. In other words, allergy came to be defined only in terms of conditions related to the body's immune system. It is claimed that immunity and allergy both stem from the same mechanism. 'Those reactions which appear to benefit the individual are considered manifestations of immunity, those that are harmful, manifestations of allergy' stated Sherman.

However, the discovery of 'food allergies' in the modern context, has shown a much wider list of symptoms which hitherto had not been considered as being 'allergic' in origin and as a result, had often been disregarded by the conventional allergists as not being appropriate to their field of study.

The orthodox allergist often appears to consider only those allergies which are visible; the skin conditions or the puffy eyes in hay fever, or the obvious manifestations of asthma. They seem almost always to relate these conditions to inhalant allergens such as pollens or house dust mite droppings; virtually no consideration is given to foods as a likely trigger. The range of disorders now being shown to be attributable to ordinary foods is a concept so far removed from their training that it almost beggars belief.

Whenever conventional allergists consider foods as being of allergenic importance, they tend to limit the likely manifestations to childhood skin conditions. They virtually never consider whether other physical or mental symptom are linked to foods.

The asthmatic, they believe, suffers as a result of an inhalant allergen. Somehow, because breathing is involved in the asthmatic's condition, the conventional allergist looks only to aeroallergens as being causative whilst it could in fact be something as seemingly innocuous as milk or bread which was responsible for the distress.

CHAPTER TWENTY-FOUR

Food Ignored

An impressive manual, written by four Allergy-Immunology Professors of Medicine, almost 1,000 pages in length, *Allergic Diseases, Diagnosis and Management* (J.P. Lippincott Company) has this to say on food allergies:

> Foods: although foods may be important in cases of infantile eczema, urticaria, angio-edema, or anaphylaxis, they are almost never important in cases of allergic conjunctivitis, allergic rhinitis, or allergic asthma. The antigens most important in those conditions are usually airborne.
>
> Several different groups of these aeroallergens are of major clinical significance, including the pollens, fungi, house dust mite, and animal danders.

This relatively recent (1993) and impressive immunologically-focussed work virtually skirts over nutrition, and ignores the vast number of other conditions which we now know can be brought on by the mere act of consuming foods or drinks, or inhaling an allergen not even commonly considered by such eminent men: ordinary gas fires, wallpaper paste, airborne fungi, or paint fumes. These have, amongst many other commonly-encountered fumes, been shown to be implicated in many health disorders other than those normally considered by the conventional allergist.

Anaphylaxis

Anaphylaxis is a serious allergic reaction which can result in obstruction to breathing. Occasionally people have died from such an attack. In 1902, Richet and Portier described the development of anaphylaxis in dogs given sea anemone toxin. Subsequently, anaphylaxis was described in humans after the injection of horse serum to achieve immunisation against tetanus and diphtheria.

In 1906, Clemons von Pirquet predicted that immunity and hypersensitivity reactions would depend on the interaction between a foreign substance and the immunologic system, and that immunity and hypersensitivity would have similar underlying immunologic mechanisms.

The search for the factor responsible for immediate hypersensitivity reactions became a subject of intense investigation over a number of years. In 1921, Prausnitz and Kustner described the transfer of immediate hypersensitivity by serum.[127]

However, as much as von Pirquet recognised that the allergic reaction resulted from the reaction between a 'foreign substance' and the immunologic system, it does little to explain why not everyone would produce symptoms of an allergic nature when exposed to similar 'foreign' (and often they are not foreign, but completely 'natural') substances.

Dr. Kustner was anaphylactically sensitive to fish protein. He and a colleague demonstrated that intradermal injection of his serum into the skin of a normal individual followed by a fixation period of 24 hours would result in a local, immediate reaction when the site of serum implantation was challenged with fish antigen. This test for the serum factor responsible for immediate hypersensitivity reactions was termed the Prausnitz-Kustner test (P-K test). Variations of this test remained the standard for measuring skin-sensitising antibody over the next 50 years.

Antibodies are special proteins which circulate in the blood and attack incoming allergens in an attempt to render them harmless. In 1925, Coca and Grove did extensive studies in the USA of the skin-sensitising factor from sera of patients with hay fever.

They called the skin-sensitising antibody atopic reagin (allergic antibody) because of its association with hereditary conditions and because of their uncertainty as to the exact nature of the factor.[128]

Many immunologists believed that this reaginic antibody in hay fever belonged to a class of immunoglobulins called IgA (IgA stands for immunoglobulin A; an immunoglobulin is one of a group of structurally related proteins that act as antibodies). IgA is a protective anitbody produced in breast milk. However, in 1967 the Ishizakas discovered that skin-sensitising antibody belonged to a unique class of immunoglobulin, which they called IgE.[129]

Further immunoglobulin types are IgG, IgM and IgD all of which have been implicated either individually or collectively in various conventionallly-considered allergic states. IgE is considered to be implicated in 'hereditary' allergic conditions such as asthma and hay fever. Immunoglobulin G (IgG) is small and is known to cross the placental barrier and is often linked with other Ig's in allergy reactions.

IgM is an immunoglobulin composed of larger molecules and although IgD is known as an immunoglobin, its function is not yet fully understood.

Whilst the presence of the above immunoglobulins is a feature of various hypersensitivity states in allergy, it is the case that their measured presence is not always seen during attacks of food allergy (see Felder study below) about which this book is written. And if their measured presence is not evident in all food allergy attacks, then it must be the case that their presence cannot be an indicator of such 'allergic' activity, which explains why blood tests for food allergies must be considered questionable at the very best.

The question must be asked therefore, just how important is the existence of any or all of these antibodies in the bloodstream, in the diagnosis of the 'food' or 'chemical' allergy about which this book is written?

If the required measured presence of any of the above antibodies in the system, directly indicated or implied the presence of an hypersensitivity state 100% of the time, then I would consider it of importance. But the food or chemical allergic state, about which this book is written, will not necessarily abide by the requirements relating to immunoglobulin presence which the orthodox allergist seeks.

Food 'allergies' not Ig mediated

Evidence that the 'unconventional' food allergy phenomenon is without the 'conventional' immunological basis which orthodox allergists expect to find, comes from one study of six patients who exhibited rheumatoid arthritis when exposed to food allergens.

Felder and others showed that six patients who were food allergic and whose symptoms were rheumatoid arthritis were investigated clinically in laboratory tests to see if there were any immunologic reactions and they reported that 'There was no sign of an immunologic reaction in any of the measured parameters.'[130]

That important study told me what I had suspected for some time, that the 'unconventional' food allergic patient is in a different medical category altogether from that in which the 'recognised' immunologically-mediated allergic condition finds itself. The masked allergy condition has no immunological-mediated basis whatsoever in my opinion, and in that of a growing number of researchers.

The food allergic syndrome about which this book refers will almost certainly not be the classically-considered IgE, IgA or even IgM-mediated allergies. The allergies about which this book is written will not be immunological in their origins – that seems certain. And thus, it will be deemed foreign to the conventional allergist who focuses heavily on IgE and other Iummoglobulin-mediated values in their work.

It is clear to me that as parasites are now implicated in the condition referred to as 'masked food allergy', these organisms appear not to invoke a true Ig response at all, being past-masters at evading the immunological defences. I think that the Ig responses picked out by food allergy blood tests do indeed identify a raised immunoglobulin presence, but, in my opinion, such Ig activity *plays no part* in the food allergic reaction, or, to put it another way, plays *no part* in the patient's symptoms.

Allergy, hypersensitivity, or intolerance?

It is a valid observation that there is an entire world of people out there suffering as a result of eating foods to which their bodies are reacting abnormally. As allergy means 'altered reaction' and as we are substantially talking about foods, then we have little alternative but to label these reactions as food allergies. There always will be the old guard however who want to label these reactions 'hypersensitivities' or 'intolerances'. If you are run over by a car it is of little consequence that it might be a red car, a blue car or a black car; you were simply run over by a car and that is all that should matter.

If you have symptoms of ill health, find a dietary connection to the symptoms, remove the culprit foods, and watch your symptoms abate or disappear as a result, it would be a foolish person who argued that some adverse reaction, some intolerance, to that substance had not been shown. Whether the 'allergy' has an immunological or non-immunological basis is unimportant if the connection has been established.

AFTERWORD

And what about my own condition, my own food 'allergies'? There's a tale to tell here. I recently went to London to buy a car, since it was considerably cheaper to buy there than where I live.

While I was in London I decided to give myself a treat and take the first break from my diet in six months. I knew a day or so off the diet would not be critical, so long as it didn't extend far beyond that.

I went to a favourite restaurant, one I had visited many times before. It was under the same ownership and I chose the meal that I always seemed to choose when I went there: nothing exotic, just plain shepherd's pie, roast potatoes and vegetables.

I love this particular meal but have always paid for it with a real flattener of a reaction. As sure as night follows day, within half an hour of starting the meal I would feel the familiar fatigue-like reaction wash over me. I could set my watch by it; the massive reaction never varied. If I went on holiday to London, or was simply passing through, I would make a point of visiting the restaurant, yet without fail would suffer as a consequence of eating that meal.

This time I became aware, half an hour or so after the meal, that no new reaction had taken place. I was still feeling a bit of a light reaction from the small hotel breakfast I had had a couple of hours before, but it was only mild.

I presumed the big reaction was running late, so to speak, perhaps because my body chemistry had changed due to the length of time I had been on a natural diet.

After three quarters of an hour I began to contemplate the impossible: that I might get away with eating this meal without any reaction at all. That would be a dream come true. I wanted to phone my daughter straight away to tell her, but thought I had better hold on just in case the reaction was still to come.

I went browsing in an antique shop, but I was more excited about the prospect of getting away with eating the meal than by what was on offer in the shop. Surely it was a false dawn? Any minute now, no doubt, a blaster of a reaction would occur!

After an hour and a half, when a reaction should have been well under way, if not wearing off again, no reaction had occurred . In fact the only change was that the mild reaction from breakfast was no longer in evidence!

This astonishing event was very, very special to me. It was a massive discovery and surely, at last, reward for following to the letter such a rigid dietary regimen.

Well, I did phone my daughter, and I didn't stop there. I phoned many other people besides, absolutely thrilled to have had such an unexpected - and it truly was unexpected - response to eating a meal well-established as allergenic; one which hitherto had always provoked a massive response in me.

I am continuing my diet, as my temperature is still showing signs of climbing and I want to go on until it has reached, and *stabilised* at, as near to 98.6 as it can. It should be expected then that the mild reactions I now sometimes get will be a thing of the past!

I hope this story will encourage you in your own endeavours.

Appendix

AUTHOR'S UPDATED TEMPERATURE CHART

Here are the author's temperature readings at the conclusion of writing this book. As you will see, the temperature pattern is climbing all the time, albeit erratically. This erratic nature of dietary recovery is to be expected, but the reward for complying with Nature's laws is that recovery, when it comes, will be lasting.

Months 1-14

1	2	3	4	5	6	7	8	9	10	11	12	13	14
0	0	0	0	0	1	2	1	2	6	5	4	6	5

Days 98.3F. degrees or higher

1	2	3	4	5	6	7	8	9	10	11	12	13	14
5	6	7	8	5	5	14	10	12	19	12	17	18	18

Days 98.0F. degrees or higher

1	2	3	4	5	6	7	8	9	10	11	12	13	14
10	12	12	16	16	16	25	21	25	26	28	28	29	28

Days 97.8F. degrees or higher

1	2	3	4	5	6	7	8	9	10	11	12	13	14
5	9	11	1	4	2	1	1	1	0	0	0	0	0

Days 97.5F. degrees or lower

Temperatures are taken under arm for 10 minutes each morning in bed, before rising. The erratic nature of body temperature 'correction' by natural means is evident from the above figures, but we now break down further these readings into 3 monthly groups (for first 12 months) and the progress of the temperature increase becomes even more remarkable:

Days	First 3 Months	Second 3 Months	Third 3 Months	Fourth 3 Months
98.3 and above	0	1	5	15
98.0 and above	18	18	36	48
97.8 and above	34	48	71	82
97.5 and below	25	7	3	0

Remember that the above 3 monthly groups of readings can only ever reach a maximum figure of approximately 90 (days in 3 months), so the 97.8 and above figure is approaching that maximum, and hence stability. So too are the lower, wholly undesirable readings of 97.5 and below; these have been entirely eliminated, which means that stability even in this area of low readings has also been achieved.

It might well be unrealistic to expect the 98.3 and above figure to ever reach the maximum 90 bearing in mind the morning reading is *not* likely to be the highest reading of the day. However from only 1 day in the first three months to 15 in the last three months itself is astonishing progress.

When you are recording your own progress, it is worthwhile every now and then to group the months together, as I have done above, to get an even clearer insight into the actual climbs being achieved.

This clear, visible progress, of such an important indicator of your health, will, more than anything, spur you on to completing the course.

A future book will contain many case histories of people who have recovered from the food/chemical allergy condition and other common illnesses by using the method contained herein.

Readers who follow the diet and recover from their health problems and wish to be considered for inclusion in the book of recoveries, please contact the author c/o the publisher.

References

1 Langer, S.E. M.D.: *Solved: The Riddle of Illness:* Keats Publishing, New Canaan, Conn USA, 1984.

2 Lou H.C., Henriksen L., Bruhn P., Borner H., Nielsen J.B.: Striatal dysfunction in attention deficit and hyperkinetic disorder: *Arch. Neurol.,* 1989, 46:46-52.

3 Seto H., Shimizu, Futatsuya R., Kageyama M., Wu Y., Kamei T, Shibata R., Kakishita M.: Basilar artery migraine. Reversible ischaemia demonstrated by Tc-99m HMPOA brain SPECT. *Clinical Nuclear Medicine.* 19(3):215-8, 1994 Mar.

4 Guariso G., Bertoli S., Cernetti R., Battistella P.A., Setari M., Zacchello F.: Migraine and food intolerance: a controlled study in pediatric patients: *Pediatria Medica e Chirurgica.* 15(1):57-61, 1993 Jan-Feb.

5 Thomsen L.L., Iversen H.K., Olsen J.: Cerebral blood flow velocities are reduced during attacks of unilateral migraine without aura. *Cephalalgia.* 15(2):109-16. 1995 Apr.

6 Olsen J., Friberg L., Olsen T.S., Andersen A.R., Lassen N.A., Hansen P.E., Karle A. Ischaemia-induced (symptomatic) migraine attacks may be more frequent than migraine-induced ischaemic insults. *Brain.* 116(Pt1):187-202, 1993 Feb.

7 Lunardi C., Bambara L.M., Biasi D., Zagnia P., Caramaschi P., Pacor M.L. Elimination diet in the treatment of selected patients with hypersensitivity vasculitis. *Clinical & Experimental Rheumatology.* 10(2):131-5, 1992 Mar-Apr.

8 Gittleman, Ann Louise: *Guess What Came to Dinner* (p39): Avery Publishing, Garden City, N.Y., 1993.

9 Duerden, B.I.: Reid, T.M.S., Jewsbury, J.M.: *Microbial and Parasitic Infection* (p180): Edward Arnold, London, 1993.

10 Charters, A.D.: *Human Parasitology* (p152): Perth, Australia, 1983.

11 Gittleman, Ann Louise: *Guess What Came to Dinner.* Avery Publishing, Garden City Park. N.Y., 1993.

12 Duerden, B.I., Reid, T.M.S., Jewsbury, J.M.: *Microbial and Parasitic Infection* (pp5-6): Edward Arnold, London, 1993.

13 Englund, Paul T., Sher, Alan: *The Biology of Parasitism*: Alan R. Liss Inc., New York, 1998, p151

14 Paparone, P.W.: Lyme Disease Center for South Jersey, Absecon, New Jersey: Hypothyroidism with concurrent Lyme Disease: *Journal of the American*

Osteopathic Association: 95(7):435-7, July 1995.

15 *News of the World*, 29/11/1998, p38.

16 Rude,R.A. et al.: Survey of Fresh Vegetables for Nematodes, Amoebae and Salmonella: *J. Assoc. Off. Anal. Chem,* vol 67, no. 3, 1984, pp 613-615.

17 Keeton,Wm T., Gould, James L., *Biological Science*: W.W. Norton Company, New York, 1967, pp1121-1122.

18 Cited in R. Buchsbaum, *Animals without Backbones,* 2nd ed; University of Chicago Press, 1948; pp 156-157.

19 Wilson, E.Denis, M.D.: *Wilson's Syndrome*: Cornerstone Publishing Company, Orlando, Florida, 1996.

20 Marshall, Noel K: *A Chilling Effect*, Psychology Today (Feb 1982: 92).

21 Milton, Anthony S. *Pyretics and Antipyretics (Handbook of Experimental Pharmacology)*: Springer-Verlag, New York, 1982, p9.

22 Duerden, Reid, Jewsbury: *Microbial and Parasitic Infection:* Edward Arnold, London 1993, p16.

23 Wilson, Alan R.: *An Introduction to Parasitology,* New York: St. Martin's Press, 1967.

24 Wilson, Alan R.: *An Introduction to Parasitology,* New York: St. Martin's Press, 1967.

25 Wilson, Alan R.: *An Introduction to Parasitology,* New York: St. Martin's Press, 1967.

26 Sun, T: *Color Atlas and Textbook of Diagnostic Parasitology*, 1988.

27 Literature: Great Smokies Diagnostic Laboratory, Asheville, North Carolina, 1998, p2.

28 Wahlgren M.: Lancet 1991: 337:675; Corcoran G.D. et al.: *Lancet*, 1991, 338:254;: Veraldi, S. et al.: *Int. J. Derm*, 1991; 30:376: RolstonK.V.I. et al. *New England Journal of Medicine*, 1986 (July 17):192.

29 Kluger, J.: Fever - New Perspectives on an Old Phenomenon: *New England Journal of Medicine:* (April 21,1983):308;16,958.

30 Milton, Anthony S.: *Pyretics and Antipyretics (Handbook of Experimental Pharmacology)*: Springer-Verlag New York, 1982.

31 Duerden, Reid, Jewsbury: *Microbial and Parasitic Infection*: Edward Arnold, London, 1993, p43.

32 Charters, A.D.:*Human Parasitology*: Perth, Australia, 1983.

33 Duerden, Reid, Jewsbury: *Microbial and Parasitic Infection*: Edward Arnold, London 1993, p145.

34 *Ibid,* p200.

35 Literature: Great Smokies Diagnostic Laboratories, Asheville, N.C., USA, 1998.

36 Charters, A.D.: *Human Parasitology*: Charters, Kalamunda, Western Australia, p70.

37 Cox, F.E.G.: *Modern Parasitology*: Blackwell Science, Oxford, England, 1993 (Lyme Disease p71).

38 Duerden, Reid, Jewsbury: *Microbial and Parasitic Infection*: Edward Arnold, London, 1993 (Salmonella, pp310-311).

39 Hawken, C.M.: *Parasites*: Woodland Publishing, Pleasant Grove, Utah, p17.

40 BBC TV, News, 6pm 14 Aug 1998.

41 Charters, A.D.: *Human Parasitology*: Charters, Kalamunda, Western Australia, p34.

42 Hawken, C.M.: *Parasites*; Woodland Publishing, Pleasant Grove, Utah, p17.

43 Literature: Great Smokies Diagnostic Laboratories, Asheville, NC, USA, 1998.

44 Charters, A.D.: *Human Parasitology:* Charters, Kalamunda, Western Australia, p34.

45 Literature: Great Smokies Diagnostic Laboratories, Asheville, N.C., USA, 1998.

46 Gittleman, Ann Louise: *Guess What Came to Dinner.* Avery Publishing, Garden City Park, N.Y., 1993, p23.

47 Chaitow, Leon: *Candida Albicans*: Thorsons, 1985, p10.

48 Hawken, C.M.: *Parasites*: Woodland Publishing, Pleasant Grove, Utah, p16.

49 Gittleman, Ann Louise: *Guess What Came to Dinner.* Avery Publishing, Garden City Park, N.Y., 1993, p46.

50 Hawken, C.M.: *Parasites*: Woodland Publishing, Pleasant Grove, Utah, p16.

51 Wilson, R. Alan: *An Introduction to Parasitology*: St. Martin's Press, New York, 1967.

52 Duerden, Reid, Jewsbury: *Microbial and Parasitic Infection*: Edward Arnold, London 1993, p141-142.

53 Duerden, Reid, Jewsbury: *Microbial and Parasitic Infection*: Edward Arnold, London 1993, p111.

54 Literature: Great Smokies Diagnostic Laboratories, Asheville, N.C., USA, 1998.

55 Charters, A.D.: *Human Parasitology*: Charters, Kalamunda, Western Australia, p122.

56 Charters, A.D.: *Human Parasitology*: Charters, Kalamunda, Western Australia, p122.

57 Gittleman, Ann Louise: *Guess What Came to Dinner.* Avery Publishing, Garden City Park, N.Y., 1993.

58 Great Smokies Diagnostic Laboratories, Asheville, N.C., USA, 1998.

59 Literature: Great Smokies Diagnostic Laboratories, Asheville, N.C., USA, 1998.

60 Duerden, Reid, Jewsbury: *Microbial and Parasitic Infection*: Edward Arnold, London 1993, p303-304.

61 Gittleman, Ann Louise: *Guess What Came to Dinner.* Avery Publishing, Garden City Park, N.Y., 1993, p46.

62 Duerden, Reid, Jewsbury: *Microbial and Parasitic Infection*: Edward Arnold, London 1993, p134.

63 *Ibid,* p307.

64 *Ibid* p76.

65 Gittleman, Ann Louise: *Guess What Came to Dinner.* Avery Publishing, Garden City Park, N.Y., 1993, p23.

66 Duerden, Reid, Jewsbury: *Microbial and Parasitic Infection*: Edward Arnold, London 1993, p200.

67 *Ibid,* p311.

68 *Ibid,* p312.

69 *Ibid,* p314.

70 *Ibid,* p314.

71 Charters, A.D.: *Human Parasitology*, Perth, Australia, p29.

72 *Ibid,* p29.

73 *Ibid,* p26.

74 *Ibid,* p26.

75 *Ibid,* p26.

76 *Ibid,* p42.

77 *Ibid,* p43

78 *Ibid,* p75.

79 *Ibid,* p78.

80 Duerden, Reid, Jewsbury: *Microbial and Parasitic Infection*: Edward Arnold, London 1993, p284-6.

81 Literature: Great Smokies Diagnostic Laboratories, Asheville, N.C., USA, 1998.

82 Chaitow, Leon: *Candida Albicans*: Thorsons, London, 1985, p10.

83 Duerden, Reid, Jewsbury: *Microbial and Parasitic Infection*: Edward Arnold, London 1993, p41.

84 Charters, A.D.: *Human Parasitology*, Perth, W.Australia, p142.

85 *Daily Mail* : Invisible Bug is Leaving Women Infertile, 8 March 1999.

86 Duerden, Reid, Jewsbury: *Microbial and Parasitic Infection*: Edward Arnold, London 1993, p116.

87 Gittleman, Ann Louise: *Guess What Came to Dinner*: Avery Publishing, Garden City Park, N.Y., 1993, p40-41.

88 Wynburn-Mason, Roger: *The Causation of Rheumatoid Disease and Many Human Cancers: A New Concept in Medicine*: Iji Publishing Company, Tokyo, 1978.

89 Gittleman, Ann Louise: *Guess What Came to Dinner*: Avery Publishing, Garden City Park, N.Y., 1993, p32.

90 Duerden, Reid, Jewsbury: *Microbial and Parasitic Infection*: Edward Arnold, London 1993, p309.

91 BBC TV, News, 6pm 14th August 1998.

92 Gelpa, A.P. and Mustafa, A., Ascaris pneumonia: *Am.J.Med.*, 1968;44:377.

93 Orihel, Thomas C., Ash, Larence R.: *Parasites in Human Tissues*: American Soc. of Clinical Pathologists, Chicago, Ill., 1995, p86.

94 Galland, L.M.D., et al.: *Journal of Nutritional Med.1*, 1990;27-31.

95 Hawken, C.M.: *Parasites*: Woodland Publishing, Pleasant Grove, Utah, 1997.

96 Cox, F.E.G.: *Modern Parasitology*: Blackwell Science, Oxford, 1999, p209.

97 Duerden, Reid, Jewsbury: *Microbial and Parasitic Infection*: Edward Arnold, London 1993, p164.

98 Duerden, Reid, Jewsbury: *Microbial and Parasitic Infection*: Edward Arnold, London 1993 p42.

99 Marshall, Noel K.: A Chilling Effect: *Psychology Today*, Feb 1982:92.

100 Marshall, Noel K.: A Chilling Effect: *Psychology Today*:,Feb 1982:92.

101 Langer, Stephen E. M.D.: *Solved: The Riddle of Illness*: Keats Publishing, USA. 1984, p36.

102 Pleshette, Janet: *Cures That Work*: Century Arrow, London, 1986.

103 Gittleman, Ann Louise: *Guess What Came to Dinner:* Avery Publishing, Garden City Park, N.Y., 1993.

104 Milton, Anthony S.: *Pyretics and Antipyretics*: Spring-Verlag, Berlin, 1982; p189-212.

105 Levanthal, R., Cheadle, R.F: *Medical Parasitology: A Self-Instructional Text*, F.A. Davis Company, Philadelphia, 1989.

106 Hawken, C.M.: *Parasites:* Woodland Publishing, Pleasant Grove, Utah, 1997.

107 Thomsen, L.L., Iversen, H.K., Olsen, J.: Cerebral blood flow velocities are reduced during attacks of unilateral migraine without aura: *Cephalalgia*. 15(2):109-16;1995.Ap.

108 Wojewodzkiej Poradni Alergologicznej, Stalowej Woli, Migraine as one of the symptoms of food allergy: *Polski Tygodnik Lekarski*: 47(3-4):89-91,1992, Jan 20-27.

109 Cox, Prof. F.E.G.: *Modern Parasitology*: Blackwell Science, Oxford, England, 1993.

110 Cox, Prof. F.E.G., *Modern Parasitology*: Blackwell Science, Oxford,1999, p209.

111 Duerden, Reid, Jewsbury: *Microbial and Parasitic Infection*: Edward Arnold, London, 1993, p41.

112 Cox, Prof. F.E.G., *Modern Parasitology*: Blackwell Science, Oxford, 1999, p40.

113 Cox, Prof. F.E.G., *Modern Parasitology*: Blackwell Science, Oxford, 1999, p37.

114 Lou H.C., Henriksen L., Bruhn ., Borner H., Nielsen J.B.: Striatal dysfunction in attention deficit and hyperkinetic disorder: *Arch. Neurol,* 1989;46:46-52.

115 Seto H., Shimizu, Futatsuya R., Kageyama M., Wu Y., Kamei T., Shibata R., Kakishita M.: Basilar artery migraine. Reversible ischaemia demonstrated by Tc-99m HMPOA brain SPECT: *Clinical Nuclear Medicine,* 19(3):215-8, 1994 Mar.

116 Guariso G., Bertoli S., Cernetti R., Battistella P.A., Setari M., Zacchello F.: Migraine and food intolerance: a controlled study in pediatric patients: *Pediatria Medica e Chirurgica,* 15(1):57-61, 1993 Jan-Feb.

117 Thomsen L.L., Iversen H.K., Olsen J.: Cerebral blood flow velocities are reduced during attacks of unilateral migraine without aura.: *Cephalalgia*. 15(2):109-16, 1995 Apr.

118 Olsen J., Friberg L., Olsen T.S., Andersen A.R., Lassen N.A., Hansen P.E., Karle A.: Ischaemia-induced (stmptomatic) migraine attacks may be more frequent than migraine-induced ischaemic insults:*Brain*. 116(Pt1):187-202, 1993 Feb.

119 Thomsen L.L., Iversen H.K., Olsen J.: Cerebral blood flow velocities are reduced during attacks of unilateral migraine without aura. *Cephalalgia.* 15(2):109-16, 1995 Apr.

120 Forman, Robert, Ph.D.: *How to Control Your Allergies*: Larchmont Books, New York, 1980.

121 Kenton, Leslie: *Raw Energy*: Century Arrow, London, 1984.

122 Pottenger, Francis: *Pottenger's Cats: A Study in Nutrition*: Price-Pottenger Nutrition Foundation, 1983.

123 Taylor, Renee: *Hunza Health Secrets*: Keats Publishing, Conn. USA, 1964.

124 Densmore, Emmet M.D.: *How Nature Heals*: Swan Sonnenschein & Co., London, 1892.

125 Shelton, Herbert: *Getting Well*, 1946.

126 Feingold, Ben F., M.D.: *Introduction to Clinical Allergy*: Charles C. Thomas, Springfield, Ill., 1973.

127 Prausnitz C., Kustner H.: Studien über überempfindlichkeit: *Centralbl. Bakteriol* 1921;86(1):160.

128 Coca A.F., Grove E.F.: Studies in hypersensitiveness: XIII. A study of atopic rea gins: *J Immunol,* 1925;10:444.

129 Ishizaka K., Ishizaka T.: Immunology of IgE mediated hypersensitivity, In: Middleton E., Reed C.E., Ellis, eds.: *Allergy principles and practice,* 2nd ed., C.V. Mosby, St. Louis, 1983:52.

130 Felder M., De Blecourt A.C., Wuthrich B.: Food allergy in patients with rheuma toid arthritis: *Clinical Rheumatology, 6*(2):181-4., 1987 Jun.

Bibliography

Pottenger's Cats, Francis M. Pottenger Jr.: Price-Pottenger Nutrition Foundation, California.

Nutrition and Health, McCarrison: The McCarrison Society, London

The Fasting Story II, Tanner, Hotema, Hanish, Carrington: Health Research, Mokelumne, Calif.

Parasites in Human Tissues, Ash and Orihel: ASCP Press, Chicago, Illinois.

Fasting For Health And Long Life, Hereward Carrington: Health Research, Mokelumne, Calif.

Be Your Own Doctor, Ann Wigmore: Avery Publishing, Wayne, New Jersey.

Microbial and Parasitic Infection, Duerden et al: Edward Arnold, London.

Mucusless Diet Healing System, Arnold Ehret: Ehret Publishing, Yonkers, New York.

Biological Science, Keeton and Gould: W.W. Norton and Company, New York.

Solved: The Riddle of Illness, Stephen E. Langer: Keats Publishing Inc. New Canaan, Connecticut.

The Fasting Cure, Upton Sinclair (1955): Health Research, Mokelumne, California.

The Healing Crisis, C. Leslie Thomson: Thomson-Kingston Publications, Edinburgh.

In Search of the Perfect Cleanse, Jason Winters: Vinton Publishing, Las Vegas, Nevada.

Allergic to Food?, Rita Greer: J. M. Dent and Sons, London.

Body, Mind and the B Vitamins, Ruth Adams and Frank Murray: Larchmont Books, New York.

The Food Depression Connection, June Roth: Contemporary Books, Chicago, Illnois.

Modern Parasitology, Edited by F.E.G. Cox: Blackwell Science, Oxford.

The Cure for all Diseases, Hulda Clark: New Century Press, San Diego, California.

The Science and Fine Art of Fasting, Herbert Shelton: ANHS, Tampa, Florida.

Atlas of Human Parasitology, Ash and Orihel: ASCP Press, Chicago, Illinois.

Getting Well, Herbert Shelton: Health Research, Mokelumne, California.

Human Nutrition and Dietetics, Garrow and James: Churchill Livingstone, Edinburgh.

Minerals, The Metabolic Mineral Workers, Erdmann and Jones: Century Press, London.

Superior Nutrition, Herbert Shelton: Willow Publishing, San Antonio, Texas.

The Diet Book, Marguerite Requa (1937): Oxford University Press, London.

Aura and Consciousness, Konstantin Korotkov: Russian Ministry of Culture, St. Petersburg, Russia.

Parasites, C.M. Hawken: Woodland Publishing, Pleasant Grove, Utah.

Health for the Millions, Herbert Shelton: ANHS, Tampa, Florida.

Guess What Came to Dinner, Ann Louise Gittleman: Avery Publishing, Garden City Park, NY.

Essentials of Parasitology, Meyer, Olsen and Schmidt: Wm. C. Brown, Dubuque, Iowa.

The Myth of Medicine, Herbert Shelton: Cool Hand Communications, Boca Raton, Florida.

Human Life, Its Philosophy and Laws, Herbert Shelton: Kessinger Publishing, Montana.

Pyretics and Antipyretics, Edited by A.S. Milton: Springer-Verlag, Heidelberg, West Germany.

Human Parasitology, Edited by A.D. Charters: , Kalamunda, Western Australia.

Clinical Pharmacology, Laurence and Bennett: Churchill Livingstone, Edinburgh.

Diet, Crime and Delinquency, Alexander Schauss: Parker House, Berkeley, California.

Nutrition and the Mind, George Watson, California.

Food Science, Nutrition and Health, Fox and Cameron: Edward Arnold, London.

Diet and Nutrition, Rudolph Ballentine: Himalayn International Institute, Honesdale, Pennsylvania.

Allergies: Disease in Disguise, Carolee Bateson-Koch: Alive Books, Burnaby, BC, Canada.

The Science and Fine Art of Natural Hygiene, Herbert Shelton: ANHS, Tampa, Florida.

Natural Hygiene, Herbert Shelton: ANHS, Tampa, Florida.

Hunza Health Secrets, Renee Taylor: Keats Publishing, New Canaan, Connecticut.

Not All In The Mind, Richard Mackarness: Pan Books, London.

The Pulse Test, Arthur F. Coca: Arco Publishing, New York.

A Cancer Therapy (Results of Fifty Cases), Max Gerson: Gerson Institute, Bonita, California.

Fasting for Renewal of Life, Herbert Shelton: Natural Hygiene Press, Chicago.

The Complete Raw Juice Therapy, Susan E. Charmine: Thorsons, London.

Cures That Work, Janet Pleshette: Century Arrow, London.

Brain Allergies, Philpott and Kalita: Keats Publishing, New Canaan, Connecticut.

Enzyme Nutrition, Edward Howell: Avery Publishing, New Jersey.

The Colon Health Handbook, Robert Gray: Emerald Publishing, Nevada.

Natural Therapeutics, (Vols. I, II and III): Henry Lindlahr: The C. W. Daniel Co., Saffron Walden.

Chemical Victims, Richard Mackarness: Pan Books, London.

Philosophy of Natural Therapeutics, Henry Lindlahr: The C. W. Daniel Co., Saffron Walden.

Nutrition and Physical Degeneration, W. A. Price: Keats Publishing, New Canaan, Connecticut.

Food in Antiquity, Don and Patricia Brothwell: Thames and Hudson, London.

How to Fortify Your Immune System, Donald Dickenson: Arlington Books, London.

Food Facts and Fallacies, Fredericks and Bailey: Arco Publishing, New York.

Nutrition and Mental Illness, Carl F. Pfeiffer: Healing Arts Press, Vermont.

Overfed but Undernourished, Curtis Wood Jr.: Tower Publications, New York.

New Hope for Incurable Diseases, Cheraskin and Ringsdorf: Arco Publishing, New York.

Nerve Troubles: Science of Life Books, Melbourne, Australia.

Dr. Schuessler's Biochemistry, J. B. Chapman: Thorsons, London.

Against the Unsuspected Enemy, Amelia Nathan Hill: New Horizon, Bognor Regis.

I Fought Leukemia - and Won!, Rex B. Eyre: Hawkes Publishing, Salt Lake City.

Feasting on Raw Foods, Edited by Charles Gerras: Thorsons, London.

Super Natural Immune Power, Weller: Thorsons, London.

Let's Eat Right to Keep Fit, Adelle Davis: Unwin Books, New York.

Let's Cook it Right, Adelle Davis: Unwin Books, New York.

Cancer? Think Curable: The Gerson Therapy, Gerson Institute, Bonita, California.

The Manual of Natural Living, Barreau and Salomon: Thorsons, London.

The Healthy Human Gut, C. Leslie Thomson: Thomson-Kingston Publications, Edinburgh.

Improve Your Sight Without Glasses, Science of Life Books: Melbourne, Australia.

Skin Troubles, Leon Chaitow: Thorsons, London.

Raw Energy, Leslie and Susannah Kenton: Arrow Books, London.

The Allergy Connection, Barbara Paterson: Thorsons, London.

Megavitamin Therapy, Ruth Adams and Frank Murray: Larchmont Books, New York.

How to Get Rid of the Poisons in Your Body, Gary and Steven Null: Arco Publishing, New York.

Homoeopathy and Your Emotions, Sheila Harrison: Ashgrove Press, Bath.

Daniel; Living With an Allergic Child, Diana Wells: Ashgrove Press, Bath.

Food for Fitness: World Publications, Mountain View, California.

Your Daily Diet, Geoffrey Whitehouse: Newman Turner Publications, London.

Let's Stay Healthy, Adelle Davis: Unwin Books, New York.

How to Live With Hypoglycemia, Charles Weller: Jove Publications, New York.

A Natural Approach; Allergies, Michio Kushi: Japan Publications, New York.

About Fasting, Otto H. F. Buchinger: Thorsons, London.

How to Live Longer and Feel Better, Linus Pauling: W. H. Freeman and Co. New York.

Nutritional Influences on Mental Illness, Melvyn R. Werbach: Third Line Press, Tarzana, California.

Anatomy and Physiology, Ross and Wilson: Churchill Livingstone, Edinburgh.

10 Day Clean-Up Plan, Leslie Kenton: Century Books, London.

Live Food Juices, H. E. Kirschner: H. E. Kirschner Publications, Monrovia, California.

Fasting: The Ultimate Diet: Alan Cott: Bantam Books, New York.

The Stone-Age Health Programme, Eaton et al.: Angus and Robertson, NSW. Australia.

Nutritional Influences on Illness, Melvyn R. Werbach: Third Line Press, Tarzana, California.

Instinctive Nutrition, Schaeffer: Celestial Arts, California.

Fasting, Shirley Ross: Sheldon Press, London.

Fasting Can Save Your Life, Herbert Shelton: ANHS Publications, Tampa, Florida.

The Miracle of Fasting, Paul C. Bragg: Health Science, Santa Barbara, California.

Candida Albicans, Leon Chaitow: Thorsons, London.

How to Control Your Allergies, Robert Forman, Larchmont Books, New York.

Cancer Winner, Jacquie Davison: Midwest Press, Pierce City, Missouri.

The Migraine Revolution, John Mansfield, Thorsons, London.

The Allergy Problem, Vicky Rippere: Thorsons, London.

A Time to Heal, Beata Bishop: Hodder and Stoughton, London.

Nutrition and Disease, Edited by R. J. Jarrett: Croom Helm, London.

Vibrant Health, Norman Walker: Norwalk Press, Arizona.

Low Blood Sugar, Martin L. Budd: Thorsons, London.

Let's Get Well, Adelle Davis: Unwin Books, New York.

Overcoming Addictions, Janet Pleshette: Thorsons, London.

The Secrets of Successful Fasting, H. Lutzner: Thorsons, London.

Psycho-Nutrition, Carlton Fredericks: Putnam Publishing, New York.

Clear Body, Clear Mind, Leon Chaitow: Unwin Paperbacks, London.

Minerals: Kill or Cure?, Adams and Murray: Larchmont Books, New York.

A Matter of Life, Coates and Jollyman: MacDonald and Co., London.

BIBLIOGRAPHY

Rational Fasting, Arnold Ehret, Ehret Publishing, Yonkers, New York.

Nutrition and Its Disorders, Donald S. McLaren: Churchill Livingstone, Edinburgh.

Mental Illness and Schizophrenia, Carl Pfeiffer: Thorsons, London.

Clinical Ecology, Lewith and Kenyon: Thorsons, London.

Become Younger, Norman Walker: Norwalk Press, Arizona.

The Shocking Truth About Water, Patricia and Paul C. Bragg: Health Science, California.

Colon Health, Norman Walker: Norwalk Press, Arizona.

The Amino Revolution, Erdmann and Jones: Century Books, London.

The Grape Cure, Joanna Brandt: Ehret Literature Co., Yonkers, New York.

Body, Mind, and Sugar, Abrahamson and Pezet: Avon Books, New York.

Fighting Depression, Harvey M. Ross: Larchmont Books, New York.

Tracking Down Hidden Food Allergies, W. G. Crook: Professional Books, Tennessee.

Raw Vegetable Juices, Norman Walker: Jove Books, New York.

Food Allergy: Provocative Testing and Injection Therapy, J. Miller: Chas. Thomas, Springfield, Ill.

Consultations

International or long-distance consultations with the author, by e-mail, fax, or telephone, can be arranged. A limited number of free, or reduced-charge, consultations are available for people in hardship. You may contact Alan Hunter at:

e-mail: foodallergycure@virginbiz.com
Fax: ++44 (0)131-447-4454
Telephone: ++44 (0)131-447-9440

USEFUL ADDRESSES

United Kingdom

Plaskett College of Nutritional Medicine
Three Quoins House
Trevallett
Launceston
Cornwall
PL15 8SJ

Tel: 01566-86118
Fax: 01566-86301

British College of Naturopathy and Osteopathy
Lief House
3 Sumpter Close
120-122 Finchley Road
London
NW3 5HR
Tel: 020-7435-6464

Keki Sidhwa N.D., D.O.,
Shalimar
Harold Grove
Frinton-on-Sea
Essex
CO13 9BD

Tel: 01255-672823
(*Fasting practitioner*)

Action Against Allergy
P.O. Box 278
Twickenham
Middlesex
TW1 4QQ

(*Charity devoted to food/chemical allergies. Promotes awareness
of the condition and sends newsletter to its members. Please
include SAE if requesting information*)

USA

Dr. Virginia Vetrano D.C., hM.D.
P.O. Box 190
Barksdale, Texas 78828-0190

Tel: 830-234-3499
Fax: 830-234-3599

(*Dr. Vetrano contributed* Tosca's Fever *to this book. A student
of world-renowned fasting expert Dr. Herbert Shelton, she
now gives physiological guidance and Hygienic
counselling by telephone*)

Dr. Hulda Clark Research Association
8135 Engineer Road
San Diego, CA 92111
Tel: 800-220-3741
Fax: 858-565-0058

The Gerson Institute
P.O. Box 430
Bonita, California 91908-0430

Tel: 619-585-7600
Fax: 619-585-7610

American Natural Hygiene Society Inc.
P.O. Box 30630
Tampa, Florida 33630

Tel: 813-855-6607
(Disseminates information on fasting etc.)

Index

– V –

– W –

Notes

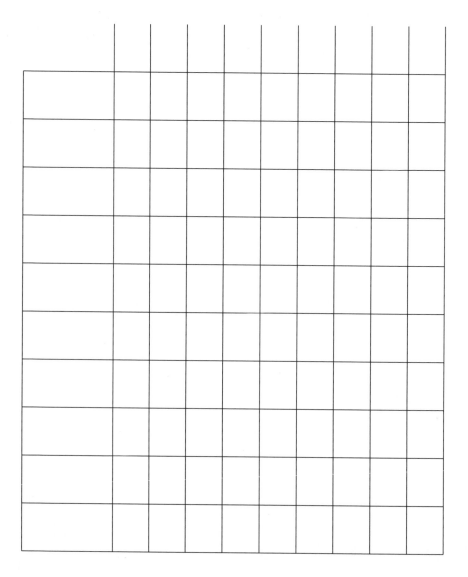

CHARTS

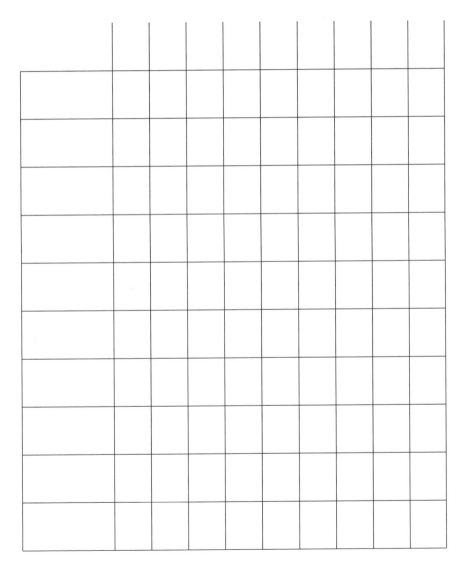

189

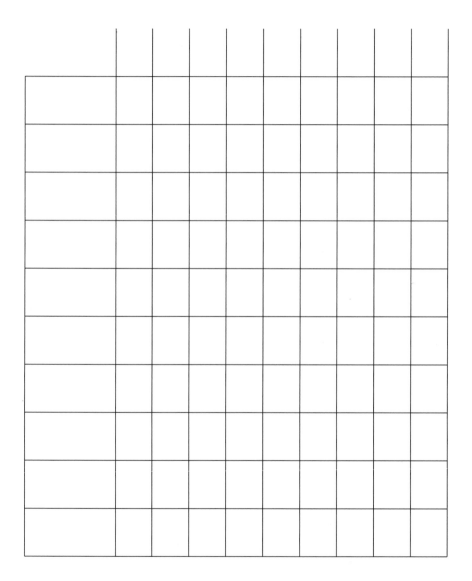

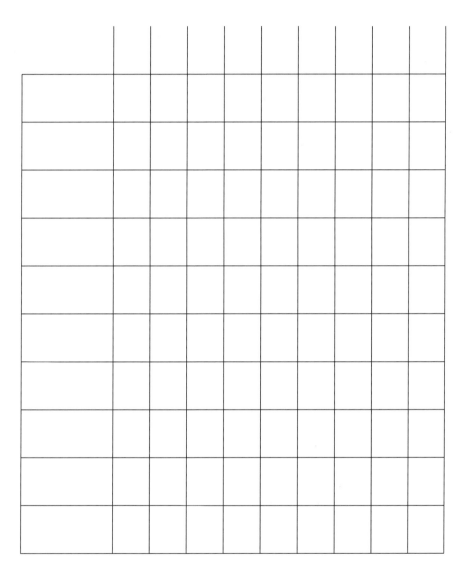

First Published in Great Britain by
ASHGROVE PUBLISHING
an imprint of
HOLLYDATA PUBLISHERS LTD
55 Richmond Avenue
London N1 0LX

First Edition

ISBN 1 85398 123 0

Printed and bound in Malta by Interprint